DMSO Healing Made Easy

Beginner's Dimethyl Sulfoxide Guide to Safe Dosage, Dilution & Topical Use for Chronic Pain, Inflammation, Joint Health, and Muscle Recovery for Natural Holistic Wellness

Amelia Hartwell

SDP Publications LLC

First edition 2026

Contents

Introduction 1

1. DMSO Basics: What It Is, How It Works, and Whether You Should Try It 5
2. How to Avoid Dangerous DMSO (And Find the Real Thing) 14
3. Safety First: Your Complete Guide to Risk-Free DMSO Use 26
4. Getting It Right: How Much DMSO to Use, How Strong, and How Often 39
5. From Arthritis to Sports Injuries: Custom DMSO Protocols for Common Conditions 60
6. Creating Custom DMSO Blends and Solving Common Problems 72
7. Advanced DMSO: What Works for Pets, What's Experimental, and What to Avoid 89
8. Getting Your Doctor on Board: How to Talk About DMSO Without Getting Dismissed 99

Printable Bonuses 111

Conclusion 113

Resources 118

Introduction

If you're reading this, there's a good chance you've had enough of pain running the show. Maybe it's a dull ache in your knee that flares up every time you climb the stairs, or your hands have started to protest after simple tasks like opening jars or typing at your desk. Perhaps you've tried creams, pills, hot packs, cold packs, and still find yourself awake at 3 a.m., scrolling through forums and blogs in search of something (anything) that might actually help.

You're not alone. I've spent years talking to people just like you: folks who are tired of the endless cycle of pain and side effects, who want relief without trading one problem for another. Many of us are looking for safer, more natural ways to feel better. We want solutions that don't come with a list of warnings longer than the directions. We want to feel in control.

That's where DMSO comes in. Maybe you've heard about it from a neighbor or a late-night internet deep dive. Dimethyl Sulfoxide (DMSO for short) has been around for decades, and its story is as fascinating as it is confusing. It's a chemical that started out as a byproduct of papermaking, then found its way into research labs, horse barns, and eventually into the hands of people desperate for relief. Along the way, it picked up all sorts of rumors and half-truths. Some call it a miracle cure. Others warn it's too dangerous to touch. And somewhere between those extremes, most of us are left wondering: what's real, and what's just hype?

I wrote this book because I've been on that same journey of questions. As someone who's passionate about helping adults overcome pain, arthritis, and inflammation, I wanted to cut through the noise and give you something real. Over the years, I've seen how confusing and overwhelming the DMSO landscape can be. One minute, you're reading a glowing review. Next, you stumble on a stern warning or conflicting "facts." It's no wonder so many people feel stuck.

So, why trust this book? For starters, I care deeply about getting things right. I believe you deserve honest, clear, and practical advice that respects both your intelligence and your safety. I've spent countless hours reading studies, talking to experts, and (most importantly) listening to people who actually use DMSO. My goal is not to sell you magic or false hope. It's to help you make informed decisions about your health, using the best knowledge available.

Here's what makes this book different: It's written for you, the beginner, who wants straightforward guidance without jargon or scare tactics. You'll find simple, step-by-step instructions for using DMSO safely. I'll walk you through when, where, and how to apply it, what to mix it with, and how to spot quality products. You'll learn how to patch test, what to do (and what not to do) with your skin, how to store DMSO, and how to avoid the most common pitfalls.

But this isn't just a "how-to" manual. You'll get real decision trees and printable checklists to help you track your progress. I'll share practical routines for joint pain, muscle soreness, headaches, and general inflammation, plus easy recipes for blends you can make at home. You'll learn how to talk to your doctor about DMSO and what to know about the legal landscape, so you're never caught off guard.

More than anything, this book puts safety first. DMSO is powerful, and it deserves respect. I'm here to encourage responsible experimentation: trying things out in small, thoughtful steps, and keeping good notes. I'll show you how to track your doses, timing, and results, so you can learn what works for you. If you're skeptical, that's healthy. I welcome your questions and your caution. We'll look at what the research says, where the gaps are, and what you might reasonably expect from DMSO.

It's important to be realistic. DMSO is not a cure-all, and it won't work the same way for everyone. Some people feel relief right away; others notice more gradual improvement. A few won't get much benefit at all. That's okay. What I want for you is clarity: knowing what you're using, why you're using it, and how to tell if it's helping. I want you to feel confident, not confused. I want you to make choices that feel right for your body and your life.

Here's how the book is set up to help you get the most out of it. The chapters are organized to guide you from the basics to hands-on routines and troubleshooting. We'll start with what DMSO is and how it works, then move into the nuts and bolts: choosing products, measuring doses, and prepping your skin. Then, we'll get specific: pain, arthritis, headaches, and more. Finally, you'll find recipes, logs, and conversation scripts to help you integrate DMSO into your life smoothly.

Throughout the book, I encourage you to take notes, jot down your questions, and track your own results. There are checklists and templates designed to make your life easier. Use them. Personalize them. Make this book a working tool, not just something you read once and put on a shelf.

So, here's my invitation: let's take back some control, one small step at a time. With the right knowledge and a healthy dose of curiosity, you can make informed choices about your pain, your health, and your well-being. You don't have to suffer in silence, and you don't have to accept "that's just how it is" as your only answer.

Ready to start? Let's get you on the path to relief, comfort, and a little more freedom in your everyday life.

Chapter One

DMSO Basics: What It Is, How It Works, and Whether You Should Try It

DMSO can seem a little confusing when you first learn about it, and it is normal to hear mixed opinions from different people. Many find relief with it, yet it helps to start with a clear understanding of what it actually is and how it works once it enters your body. With a simple, down-to-earth explanation, you can feel more comfortable as you explore whether it might be right for your own needs. A little clarity can go a long way in helping you move forward with confidence.

What Is DMSO? Understanding the Science Without the Jargon

The Basics: What DMSO Actually Is

DMSO stands for dimethyl sulfoxide. I know that sounds intimidating, but it's really not that complicated. At its core, DMSO is an organic sulfur compound. Think of it as a simple chemical made up of carbon, hydrogen, sulfur, and oxygen atoms arranged in a specific way.

It was first isolated in the late 1800s as a byproduct of the wood pulp industry, but it didn't get much attention until the 1960s when researchers started exploring its medical potential.

Pure DMSO looks a lot like water. It's clear, colorless, and has a slightly oily feel. It mixes easily with water, which makes it versatile for different formulations. One thing people notice right away is the smell. When DMSO is absorbed through your skin or metabolized in your body, it can produce a garlic-like odor on your breath and skin. This is completely normal and harmless, but it's worth knowing about upfront so you're not surprised.

What makes DMSO special is how easily it soaks into your skin. Most creams sit on top or absorb slowly over time. DMSO penetrates quickly and deeply, carrying other substances with it. This penetration ability is both its greatest strength and the reason you need to be careful about what's on your skin when you apply it.

Where DMSO Is Used Legally: FDA Approval and Off-Label Applications

In the United States, the FDA has approved DMSO for exactly one thing: treating interstitial cystitis, a painful bladder condition. For this use, doctors instill a 50% DMSO solution directly into the bladder through a catheter. It's an established medical treatment that's been used for decades with good results.

You might be thinking, "Just one approved use?" But this is actually a big deal. It means DMSO underwent rigorous testing and review for safety and effectiveness. The FDA doesn't hand out approvals lightly. Having even one approved medical use establishes DMSO as a legitimate pharmaceutical agent, not some unproven folk remedy.

Now here's where it gets interesting. People have been using DMSO off-label for decades. Off-label just means using a medication for something other than its officially approved purpose. This happens all the time in medicine. Doctors prescribe medications off-label when they have good reason to believe the medication will help, even if that specific use hasn't been formally approved.

Off-label doesn't mean illegal or even unproven. Lots of medications get used off-label based on what doctors observe in practice, smaller studies, or a logical extension of known effects. For DMSO, people use it topically (on the skin) for arthritis, muscle pain, sports injuries, inflammation, and various other conditions. These uses don't have FDA approval, but they're legal and supported by varying amounts of research and anecdotal evidence.

DMSO has an interesting history. Back in the 1960s and 1970s, researchers got really excited about it. Studies suggested it could help with everything from arthritis to head injuries. Then came safety concerns, particularly around eye damage in animals given very high doses. The FDA put a hold on most DMSO research in the United States, which essentially froze progress for years. Research continued in other countries, especially Russia and Eastern Europe, but American medicine largely moved on.

DMSO's Place in Natural and Integrative Medicine

Even without broad FDA approval, DMSO has a dedicated following in natural health circles. Why? Because many people report that it works for them, and it aligns with preferences for topical treatments over oral medications, natural or naturally-derived substances, and therapies with relatively few side effects.

This puts DMSO in a no-man's-land. You'll find passionate supporters and harsh critics. Some doctors are open to discussing it; others dismiss it out of hand. You'll find it sold in health food stores, online supplement retailers, and veterinary supply catalogs. It exists in this gray zone between conventional medicine and alternative health.

Interestingly, vets use DMSO all the time. It's common for treating horses, especially for leg injuries and joint inflammation. Veterinary DMSO is widely accepted and well-established. Many horse owners and trainers swear by it.

The veterinary acceptance actually matters. Animals don't get placebo effects, yet DMSO consistently shows benefits in veterinary use. This suggests the effects are real, not just psychological. It also means there's a long track record of practical use, even if the applications are technically off-label for humans.

Why DMSO Remains Controversial

So if DMSO works, why isn't every doctor recommending it? The answer is complicated.

First, most DMSO research is old. Modern medicine really wants recent, large clinical trials. DMSO has plenty of older studies from the 1960s through 1980s, but few recent, large-scale randomized controlled trials. This makes it hard for doctors trained to rely on current evidence-based medicine to feel comfortable recommending it.

Second, that garlic smell is a real problem in medical settings. It sounds silly, but it's a practical barrier. Imagine a doctor's office where patients regularly smell like garlic. It affects everyone in the waiting room and makes blinding studies (where researchers don't know who got the treatment) nearly impossible.

Third, some enthusiasts have made wild claims that go way beyond the evidence. When people say DMSO cures cancer or reverses Alzheimer's, they hurt DMSO's credibility. Responsible advocates stick to what's actually supported by evidence and experience, but the over-the-top claims give everyone pause.

Finally, there's tension between what doctors are trained to recommend (FDA-approved treatments with tons of data) and what patients want to try. When someone comes in asking about DMSO, many doctors aren't sure how to respond. They don't want to dismiss a patient's interest, but they also don't want to recommend something they're not familiar with.

Understanding this controversy helps you make better decisions. You're not choosing between "real medicine" and "quackery." You're navigating a gray area where a substance has some legitimate uses, some promising research, a lot of anecdotal support, and not enough modern clinical trials to satisfy everyone.

How DMSO Works: The Penetration Power and Draw-Through Effect

Now that you know what DMSO is, let's talk about how it actually works in your body. This is where things get interesting and why DMSO requires special handling.

DMSO's Superpower: Penetrating Skin and Membranes

The most important thing to understand about DMSO is this: it goes through your skin as almost nothing else does. Your skin is designed to be a barrier. It keeps the outside world out and your inside world in. That's great for protection, but it makes it hard to deliver medications where you want them.

DMSO disrupts this barrier temporarily. Its molecular structure allows it to slip between skin cells and carry along whatever else is dissolved in it. This is called penetration enhancement, and DMSO is one of the most effective penetration enhancers known.

But here's where it gets even more interesting. DMSO doesn't just carry itself through your skin. It carries other substances with it. This property is called the "draw-through effect." If you dissolve something in DMSO and apply it to your skin, the DMSO pulls that substance through your skin along with it.

This matters a lot. If you have dirt, lotion, perfume, or anything else on your skin and then apply DMSO, you could potentially drive those substances deeper into your tissue than they'd normally go. That's why cleaning your skin before DMSO application isn't just a suggestion. It's essential for safety.

Understanding Bioavailability in Plain English

Bioavailability is just a fancy word for how much of a substance actually gets into your system and how quickly. When you swallow a pill, it has to survive your stomach acid, get absorbed through your intestinal wall, pass through your liver (which might break some of it down), and then finally reach your bloodstream. By the time all that happens, you might only get a fraction of what you swallowed.

DMSO's bioavailability is high, especially when applied to skin. It gets absorbed quickly and starts working within minutes to hours. When you apply it topically, it enters your system both locally (at the application site) and systemically (throughout your body). Some stays concentrated where you applied it; some gets carried through your bloodstream to other areas.

You can use DMSO in different ways. Most people apply it topically, putting it directly where they want relief. Some medical uses involve other routes, like the bladder instillation I mentioned earlier. You should never drink DMSO. The industrial-grade product contains impurities that make it unsafe to ingest, and even pharmaceutical-grade DMSO isn't meant to be taken orally without medical supervision.

For most people reading this book, topical application is the way to go. It's safer, easier to control, and targets the area where you need relief without unnecessarily exposing your whole system.

What DMSO Does: Anti-Inflammatory, Pain Relief, and Antioxidant Properties

So DMSO gets through your skin efficiently. But what does it actually do once it's there?

First, it reduces inflammation. When you have an injury or arthritis, your body releases chemicals called inflammatory mediators. These cause swelling, redness, heat, and pain. DMSO interferes with some of these inflammatory processes, helping to calm down the inflammatory response. This is why people use it for arthritis and injuries.

Second, DMSO relieves pain. It works partly by reducing inflammation (less inflammation means less pain), but it also has a mild numbing effect. Some people describe a cooling or tingling sensation when they apply it. The pain relief can be significant for some people and subtle for others. It varies.

Third, DMSO acts as an antioxidant. It helps scavenge free radicals, which are unstable molecules that can damage cells and contribute to inflammation and aging. By neutralizing some of these free radicals, DMSO may provide protective effects beyond just pain relief.

All of this comes from real research, not just stories. Studies have measured these effects in laboratory settings and in people. The effects are real and documented, even if they're not fully understood or universally accepted in mainstream medicine.

Why DMSO's Properties Require Special Handling

Here's the thing about DMSO's unique abilities: they cut both ways. The same property that makes DMSO effective (penetrating skin and carrying things with it) is also what makes it potentially risky if used carelessly.

If DMSO can carry beneficial substances through your skin, it can carry harmful ones too. Dirt, bacteria, chemicals from lotions or cosmetics, pesticide residues, anything on your skin can potentially get driven deeper into your tissue. This is why preparation is so important. You need clean skin, clean hands, and clean application tools.

You also need to be careful about what DMSO itself contains. Industrial-grade DMSO might have contaminants from the manufacturing process. These could include heavy metals, organic solvents, or other impurities you definitely don't want absorbed into your body. That's why pharmaceutical-grade or medical-grade DMSO is essential. The purity matters.

Concentration matters too. Pure DMSO is powerful stuff. Most people need to dilute it with water or another carrier to avoid skin irritation. We'll talk about specific dilutions later, but the key point is that more concentrated isn't necessarily better. Finding the right concentration for your skin and your condition is important.

Understanding how DMSO works helps you respect it. It's not just another cream you can slap on without thinking. It requires some care and attention. But when used properly, it's a powerful tool for managing pain and inflammation.

Is DMSO Safe for You? Who Can Use It and Who Should Avoid It

DMSO isn't for everyone. Before you start using it, you need to honestly assess whether it's appropriate for your situation.

Who Can Safely Use DMSO

If you're a generally healthy adult looking for relief from pain, arthritis, or inflammation, you're probably a good candidate for DMSO. Most people tolerate it well when they use a pharmaceutical-grade product properly diluted and applied to clean skin.

DMSO works particularly well for joint pain from arthritis, muscle aches from exercise or injury, inflammation from sports injuries, chronic pain conditions that haven't responded well to other treatments, and soft tissue injuries.

The key phrase is "generally healthy adult." That means you don't have serious underlying health conditions that would make DMSO risky, you're not taking medications that could interact badly with DMSO, your liver and kidneys are functioning normally, and you don't have conditions that affect how your body processes chemicals.

Who Should Absolutely Avoid DMSO

There are certain people who should not use DMSO at all. If you fall into any of these categories, this isn't the right treatment for you.

Pregnant or breastfeeding women should avoid DMSO completely. We don't have enough safety data about how it affects developing babies or whether it passes into breast milk in significant amounts. The risk just isn't worth it when there are safer alternatives available.

Children should not use DMSO. Most safety research has been done on adults, and we don't know enough about how DMSO affects growing bodies. Until there's better data on pediatric use, keep DMSO away from kids.

People with severe liver or kidney disease need to avoid DMSO. Your liver and kidneys process and eliminate DMSO from your body. If these organs aren't working well, DMSO could build up to harmful levels or put extra strain on already compromised organs.

If you have a known sulfur allergy, DMSO is off the table. Since DMSO contains sulfur compounds, using it when you're allergic to sulfur could trigger a serious allergic reaction. This is non-negotiable.

People with certain skin conditions should be very cautious or avoid DMSO entirely. If you have active eczema, psoriasis, open wounds, infections, or severely compromised skin barrier function where you want to apply DMSO, you need to wait until your skin has healed. DMSO on broken skin can cause severe irritation and potentially drive bacteria deeper into tissue.

Understanding Drug Interactions and Health Conditions

Even if you're not in the "absolutely no" category, you still need to think about drug interactions and existing health conditions.

If you take blood thinners like warfarin or aspirin, DMSO could potentially increase their effects. DMSO has mild blood-thinning properties of its own. When combined with anticoagulant medications, there's a theoretical risk of increased bleeding. You need to talk to your doctor before using DMSO if you're on these medications.

People taking corticosteroids like prednisone should also be cautious. DMSO might enhance the absorption of topical steroids or interact with systemic steroids in ways we don't fully understand. If you're on steroid medications, get medical advice before adding DMSO.

If you use insulin or other diabetes medications, be aware that DMSO might affect how your body processes these drugs. There's not a ton of data on this interaction, but the penetration enhancement could theoretically alter insulin absorption if you're applying DMSO near injection sites. Monitor your blood sugar carefully if you decide to use DMSO.

The bottom line: if you take any prescription medications regularly, you need to research potential interactions and ideally talk to a doctor or pharmacist who can review your specific medication list. Don't assume everything is fine just because DMSO is available without a prescription.

A Self-Assessment Guide

Here's a simple way to assess your suitability for DMSO use. Ask yourself these questions honestly:

- Am I pregnant, breastfeeding, or trying to conceive? If yes, DMSO isn't for you right now.

- Am I under 18 years old? If yes, DMSO isn't appropriate.
- Do I have severe liver or kidney disease? If yes, DMSO could be dangerous. Don't use it.
- Do I have a known sulfur allergy? If yes, avoid DMSO completely.
- Do I have active skin conditions, open wounds, or infections where I want to apply DMSO? If yes, wait until your skin has healed completely.
- Am I taking blood thinners, corticosteroids, insulin, or other medications that might interact? If yes, research interactions thoroughly and talk to a healthcare provider before using DMSO.
- Do I have diabetes, immune system problems, or other chronic health conditions? If yes, be extra cautious and consider getting medical advice before starting DMSO.

If you answered "no" to all these questions, you're probably a reasonable candidate for trying DMSO carefully. If you answered "yes" to any of them, you need to either avoid DMSO or get professional medical guidance before proceeding.

The goal isn't to scare you away from DMSO. It's to help you use it safely and appropriately. Most healthy adults can use it without problems when they follow proper protocols. But knowing your limitations and risk factors matters. Being honest with yourself about whether DMSO is right for you is the first step toward safe, effective use.

Chapter Two

How to Avoid Dangerous DMSO (And Find the Real Thing)

DMSO can offer real relief, yet the benefits only come when you choose a product that is truly safe and pure. Some bottles on the market contain impurities that can be harmful, so it helps to know what to look for before you buy anything. By learning the rules in your country and getting familiar with trustworthy suppliers, you can protect yourself from low-quality products. With a little clarity and guidance, it becomes much easier to choose DMSO you can use with confidence.

Is DMSO Legal Where You Live?

Before you buy or use DMSO, you need to understand the legal landscape where you live. The rules vary significantly from country to country, and regulations can change over time. The information in this section reflects the legal status as of 2026. Always verify current regulations in your specific location before purchasing or using DMSO.

Where DMSO Is Legal (And Where It's Not)

United States: The FDA has approved DMSO for one specific medical use, treating interstitial cystitis. For this approved use, doctors prescribe RIMSO-50, which is instilled into the bladder under medical supervision. For any other use, DMSO is not FDA-approved. However, it's not illegal to purchase or use. You can legally buy DMSO from various suppliers. The key is buying pharmaceutical-grade or USP-grade DMSO, not industrial-grade products. Veterinary DMSO is widely available because it's FDA-approved for treating horses. Some people purchase veterinary-grade

DMSO for personal use. While not illegal, ensure the product meets pharmaceutical-grade purity standards (99.9% or higher) and comes with proper documentation.

Canada: Health Canada has approved DMSO for specific medical conditions, including interstitial cystitis and certain other genitourinary conditions. DMSO maintains prescription status when sold for these approved uses. DMSO is also available in Canada as a licensed natural health product for topical use in musculoskeletal conditions. Products with a Natural Product Number (NPN) can be sold over the counter. Health Canada's Personal Importation Policy allows individuals to import small quantities of health products for personal use, though restrictions apply. The safest approach is to purchase products with proper licensing (prescription or NPN) or consult your healthcare provider.

United Kingdom: In the UK, DMSO is not licensed as a medicine for human use, with limited exceptions. However, it's not banned. You can purchase DMSO from suppliers for personal use. The MHRA doesn't regulate DMSO as a medicine unless it's marketed with medical claims. This means suppliers can sell it, and you can buy it, as long as no unapproved medical claims are made. Purchase pharmaceutical-grade DMSO from reputable sources, not industrial solvents meant for laboratory use.

Australia: Australia's TGA has not approved DMSO for general medical use. However, DMSO is not a prohibited substance, so it's not illegal to possess or use it for personal purposes. The TGA's Personal Importation Scheme permits individuals to import up to a three-month supply of certain therapeutic goods for personal use. DMSO can be imported under this scheme. Keep quantities within allowed limits and maintain proper documentation to avoid customs issues.

What 'Off-Label Use' Really Means

When a doctor prescribes an FDA-approved medication for a use other than what it was officially approved for, that's off-label prescribing. This is completely legal and quite common. When you use DMSO topically for arthritis or muscle pain (outside of a prescription scenario), you're engaging in self-directed use of a legally available substance. This is generally legal in most places, with the understanding that you're taking personal responsibility.

Self-directed use means you don't have the same medical oversight you'd get with a prescription medication. This is why education and caution are so important.

Can You Import DMSO? What You Need to Know

If pharmaceutical-grade DMSO isn't easily available locally, you might consider importing it. Most countries allow individuals to import small quantities for personal use. First, verify the product is legal in your country. Second, keep quantities reasonable. Importing a year's supply might raise red flags. Stick to a few months' worth at most. Third, proper documentation matters. Legitimate suppliers provide certificates of analysis, safety data sheets, and clear labeling. Keep this documentation with your shipment and save copies for your records. Check your country's customs regulations and follow them honestly. Most customs agencies are reasonable about personal-use quantities of legal products.

How to Buy DMSO Without Breaking the Law

In most English-speaking countries, you can legally obtain and use pharmaceutical-grade DMSO for personal use. The key is doing it right. Verify DMSO is legal in your specific location and check for recent regulatory changes. Search for "DMSO legal status [your country]" and check official regulatory websites. Only buy from suppliers who clearly state their DMSO is pharmaceutical-grade or USP-grade and provide proper documentation. Avoid suppliers who make dramatic medical claims. If a website claims "DMSO cures cancer," that's a red flag. Keep records by saving receipts, certificates of analysis, and supplier communications. When in doubt, consult with a healthcare provider or attorney familiar with health product regulations.

Quick-Reference Legal Status Guide (As of 2026)

Country | Legal Status | Personal Use | Notes

United States | FDA-approved for interstitial cystitis only | Legal to purchase and use for other purposes | Veterinary DMSO is widely available

Canada | Approved for specific conditions; available as a natural health product (NPN) | Can purchase with NPN or import small quantities | Check for Natural Product Number on packaging

United Kingdom | Not licensed as medicine for general use | Legal to purchase and use personally | Not regulated as medicine unless medical claims are made

Australia | Not TGA-approved; not prohibited | Can import up to a 3-month supply | Keep documentation; stay within import limits

Important for All Regions: Must be pharmaceutical-grade for human use. Industrial DMSO is not appropriate. Keep documentation. Follow import regulations. Regulations can change, so verify the current status.

Finding DMSO You Can Trust

Medical Grade vs. Industrial Grade: What's Safe for Human Use?

Not all DMSO is created equal. In fact, using the wrong type can be genuinely dangerous. This section will help you understand the critical differences between pharmaceutical-grade and industrial-grade DMSO, and why choosing the right type is non-negotiable.

The main difference between pharmaceutical-grade and industrial-grade DMSO comes down to purity. Pharmaceutical-grade DMSO (also called medical-grade or USP-grade) is typically 99.9% pure or higher. That remaining 0.1% or less consists of water and trace amounts of tested, safe substances. Industrial-grade DMSO, used in manufacturing and research labs, may contain various contaminants, including heavy metals, residual solvents from production, pesticides, and other impurities. These contaminants exist because industrial DMSO doesn't undergo the same rigorous purification and testing. No one is checking whether it's safe to put on your skin or absorb into your body because that's not what it's designed for.

Here's the critical part: DMSO is a powerful penetration enhancer. It doesn't just absorb through your skin. It carries other substances with it. If your DMSO contains contaminants, those contaminants go into your body, too. This is why pharmaceutical-grade purity is essential. When you use DMSO on your skin, you're not just getting DMSO. You're getting DMSO plus whatever else is in the bottle. With pharmaceutical-grade DMSO, that "whatever else" is water and tested trace substances. With industrial DMSO, it could be heavy metals, solvents, or other harmful chemicals.

The 3-Second Label Check That Could Save Your Health

Look for specific indicators when buying DMSO. The product label should explicitly state pharmaceutical-grade, medical-grade, or USP-grade. If the label only says "pure DMSO" or "99% DMSO," that's not specific enough. Purity percentage should be clearly stated as 99.9% or higher. Some products claim 99.99% or even 99.995%, which is excellent, but 99.9% is the minimum for safe use.

The supplier should provide a Certificate of Analysis (COA) for each batch. This document, issued by an independent testing laboratory, verifies the purity and safety of that specific batch. We'll discuss COAs in detail later, but for now, know that any supplier refusing to provide one should be avoided. Look for clear statements about intended use. Pharmaceutical-grade DMSO should indicate it's suitable for topical application or medical use. Industrial solvents will often state "for laboratory use only" or "not for human use."

Your Pre-Purchase DMSO Safety Checklist

Before you buy any DMSO product, verify ALL of these:

☐ Label clearly states "Pharmaceutical Grade," "Medical Grade," or "USP Grade"
☐ Purity is listed as 99.9% or higher
☐ Product has a visible batch or lot number
☐ Supplier provides or offers a Certificate of Analysis (COA)
☐ Label indicates "for topical use" or "for medical use"
☐ NO warnings that say "for industrial use only"
☐ NO warnings that say "for laboratory use only"
☐ NO warnings that say "not for human use"
☐ Supplier has clear contact information (phone, address)
☐ Price is comparable to other pharmaceutical-grade products (not suspiciously cheap)

If even ONE item is missing or unclear, do NOT purchase. Find a different supplier.

Red Flags: Warning Signs of Low-Quality Products

Price can be revealing. If DMSO is dramatically cheaper than other pharmaceutical-grade options, ask why. Quality testing and purification cost money. Rock-bottom prices often mean corners were cut somewhere. Vague or missing documentation is a serious red flag. Legitimate suppliers readily provide safety data sheets and certificates of analysis. If a supplier hesitates or refuses, walk away. Generic packaging without detailed labeling suggests the product wasn't manufactured with human use in mind. Pharmaceutical-grade products come with comprehensive labels including batch numbers, expiration dates, storage instructions, and safety information. Claims that seem too good to be true probably are. If a website promises DMSO will cure everything from cancer to the common cold, they're either lying or selling something that isn't actually DMSO. Reputable suppliers focus on factual information about purity and proper use.

Suppliers with no contact information or only an email address raise concerns. Legitimate businesses provide phone numbers, physical addresses, and clear customer service channels. Finally, if the product is labeled "for research purposes only" or "not for human consumption," believe them. These labels exist because the product doesn't meet pharmaceutical standards.

How to Research DMSO Brands Yourself

Rather than recommending specific brands (which can change in quality over time or become unavailable), here's how to evaluate any DMSO brand you're considering. This process works whether you're in the US, Canada, the UK, Australia, or elsewhere.

Start by searching for the brand name plus "DMSO reviews" and "DMSO quality." Look for reviews on independent forums, health communities, and retail sites. Pay attention to recurring themes. Multiple people mentioning the same issue is significant. Single glowing reviews or single negative reviews could be outliers or fake. Look for patterns across many reviews.

Check the manufacturer's website thoroughly. Professional pharmaceutical suppliers provide detailed product information, manufacturing processes, testing procedures, and quality control measures. They should clearly display their certifications (GMP, ISO, FDA registration, if applicable). Be wary of websites that focus more on marketing hype than technical specifications. Legitimate suppliers know their customers care about purity and documentation.

Search for the brand on regulatory warning lists. In the US, check the FDA's warning letters database. In Canada, check Health Canada's advisories. In the UK and Australia, check the MHRA and TGA warning lists, respectively. If a brand has been warned or cited for quality issues, that's a deal-breaker.

Contact the supplier directly with specific questions. Ask for their most recent Certificate of Analysis. Ask about their testing procedures. Ask about the source of their DMSO and purification methods. Reputable suppliers answer these questions readily and knowledgeably. Evasive answers or reluctance to provide documentation tells you everything you need to know.

Compare pricing across multiple suppliers. If you find pharmaceutical-grade DMSO prices ranging from $20 to $30 for a certain volume, and one supplier offers it for $8, that's suspicious. You're not looking for the cheapest option. You're looking for reasonable pricing that reflects proper manufacturing and testing costs. The most expensive isn't always the best, but the cheapest is almost certainly not pharmaceutical-grade.

Check for longevity and reputation. Companies that have been selling pharmaceutical-grade DMSO for five, ten, or fifteen years have a track record. Brand-new operations aren't automatically bad, but established companies with histories of satisfied customers are lower risk.

Look for transparency about sourcing. Some suppliers disclose where their DMSO is manufactured, whether it's from wood pulp processing or petroleum sources, and what purification methods are used. This level of transparency suggests they have nothing to hide and take quality seriously.

Verifying Quality: USP and GMP Standards Explained

USP grade means the product meets United States Pharmacopeia standards for purity, quality, and consistency. This is the gold standard for pharmaceutical-grade DMSO in the United States. EP (European Pharmacopoeia) or BP (British Pharmacopoeia) are equivalent standards in Europe and the UK, respectively. Products meeting these standards have undergone rigorous testing and quality control.

GMP certification indicates the manufacturer follows Good Manufacturing Practices (standardized procedures for quality control in pharmaceutical manufacturing). While GMP doesn't specifically certify the DMSO itself, it shows the facility maintains high standards. ISO certifications (such as ISO 9001 for quality management) demonstrate systematic quality control processes. These certifications don't guarantee purity, but they indicate the manufacturer takes quality seriously.

Be wary of vague claims like "pharmaceutical quality" without specifying which standard (USP, EP, BP). Real certifications come with documentation and can be verified. If a supplier claims certifications, you should be able to confirm them through independent sources or the documentation they provide.

Reading the Fine Print: How Labels, Safety Sheets, and Test Results Protect You

Reading Product Labels: What Actually Matters

A proper DMSO label should tell you everything you need to know at a glance. The product name and grade should be prominent, something like "Pharmaceutical Grade DMSO" or "USP Grade Dimethyl Sulfoxide." The purity percentage must be clearly stated, ideally 99.9% or higher. Each product should have a unique batch number, allowing you to trace that specific production run and match it to test results.

The expiration date tells you how long the product remains at its stated purity when stored properly.

Storage instructions should recommend storing in a cool, dry place away from light, in a sealed container. Manufacturer information should include the company name and contact information. Warning and safety information should cover skin contact, proper dilution, and keeping away from children.

Safety Data Sheets: Your Chemical Roadmap

A Safety Data Sheet (SDS) is a standardized document providing detailed information about a chemical substance. You should be able to find it on the supplier's website or request it directly. Any reputable supplier will provide this without hesitation. An SDS is divided into sections. You don't need to read the whole thing, but certain sections are particularly useful.

Section 1 (Identification) tells you the product name, manufacturer, and recommended uses. Verify this matches what you're buying. Section 3 (Composition Information on Ingredients) is critical. For pharmaceutical-grade DMSO, you should see DMSO listed at 99.9% or higher, with water making up most of the remaining percentage. Section 8 (Exposure Controls Personal Protection) gives guidance on safe handling, including protective equipment and ventilation.

What an SDS reveals about quality: If the SDS lists purity lower than the label claims, you've caught a discrepancy. If it lists concerning contaminants beyond trace water, that's a red flag. If the supplier can't or won't provide an SDS, question whether they're legitimate.

Certificates of Analysis: Your Quality Verification Tool

A Certificate of Analysis (COA) is the most important document for verifying DMSO quality. It's a report from an independent testing laboratory showing actual test results for a specific batch of DMSO. Every batch of pharmaceutical-grade DMSO should have a COA. Reputable suppliers either include it with your purchase or make it readily available.

Here's what a good COA includes: Product identification with the batch or lot number matching your product. Purity testing results showing the percentage of DMSO (you want 99.9% or higher). Residual solvent testing to check for leftover manufacturing chemicals, which should be at safe, minimal levels or non-detectable. Heavy metals testing for contaminants like lead, mercury, arsenic, and cadmium (results should show these are non-detectable or far below safety limits). Microbial testing to ensure the product isn't contaminated with bacteria.

The COA should also include testing laboratory information, including the lab's name and accreditation (the lab should be independent and properly accredited), test dates showing when the analysis was performed, and authorized signatures from the lab verifying the results.

How to Spot a Fake or Incomplete COA

Not all COAs are legitimate. Watch for these red flags: Missing dates (a legitimate COA always has test dates and issue dates). No laboratory information, or using a vague lab name you can't verify. Results that are too perfect (real testing shows slight variations; if every measurement is exactly perfect with no variation, it might be fabricated). Blank fields or incomplete testing where sections say "not tested" (question why). Poor formatting or obvious typos, since professional laboratories produce clean, professional documents. No way to verify the lab's accreditation (you should be able to look up the testing laboratory and confirm they're legitimate). Finally, if the batch number doesn't match your product, the COA is only valid for the specific batch listed.

Your 9-Step DMSO Safety Verification Process

Here's a simple process to verify your DMSO is safe. Check the label against the product description you ordered, verifying that grade, purity, and intended use match. Look for the batch number on the label. Request or download the Certificate of Analysis for that batch number. Verify the batch number on the COA matches your product. Check the purity percentage on the COA (it should be 99.9% or higher). Review contaminant testing to ensure heavy metals and residual solvents are minimal or non-detectable. Verify the testing laboratory is legitimate by doing a quick online search of the lab name. If anything doesn't match or looks suspicious, contact the supplier for clarification. If the supplier can't address your concerns, don't use the product and return it if possible.

This might seem like work for your first purchase, but once you find a reliable supplier with good documentation, reordering becomes much simpler.

Why You Should Never Throw Away Your DMSO Paperwork

Save all your DMSO documentation: labels (take a photo before opening), Safety Data Sheets, Certificates of Analysis, and purchase receipts. This documentation helps you reorder the same quality product later, provides information for healthcare providers, gives you recourse if there's a quality issue, and is useful if you face questions about importing or possessing DMSO.

Store this documentation digitally. Take photos or scan documents and keep them in a folder on your computer or cloud storage. Now that you understand how to verify product quality through documentation, let's move on to proper storage practices to keep your DMSO safe and effective.

Storing DMSO Safely: Protecting Your Investment

You've purchased high-quality pharmaceutical-grade DMSO. Now you need to store it properly to maintain its purity and safety. Poor storage can degrade DMSO, contaminate it, or create safety hazards.

The 5 Rules of Safe DMSO Storage

Store DMSO in a cool, dry place away from heat sources and direct sunlight. Room temperature is fine. A cabinet or closet away from windows works well. Keep DMSO away from light. While DMSO won't break down rapidly, darkness helps preserve quality. Amber or opaque bottles provide extra protection. If your DMSO came in a clear bottle, store it in a dark cabinet.

Ensure containers are airtight. DMSO is hygroscopic, meaning it absorbs moisture from the air. When exposed to air, DMSO pulls in water, gradually diluting itself. Always seal bottles tightly after each use. Keep DMSO in its original container when possible. If you transfer it, use only appropriate containers. Store DMSO separately from other chemicals or medications. Give it its own dedicated storage space.

Choosing the Right Containers

Not all containers are safe for storing DMSO. Glass is the best choice. It's non-reactive and won't leach anything into DMSO. Amber glass bottles are ideal because they provide light protection. HDPE plastic (high-density polyethylene) is also safe. This is the type used in milk jugs and many pharmaceutical bottles. Check the recycling symbol. HDPE is marked with a 2 inside the recycling triangle.

Never use metal containers for DMSO, as DMSO can react with metals, potentially leaching metal ions into your product. Avoid PVC plastic, polystyrene, and other plastic types. DMSO can dissolve or degrade these materials. Don't reuse food containers for DMSO storage. Food residues could contaminate your DMSO, and storing DMSO in something that looks like food creates a poisoning risk.

Don't Make These 4 Dangerous Storage Mistakes

Never store DMSO in unlabeled containers. Label clearly with "DMSO," purity percentage, date, and warnings like "For External Use Only" and "Keep Away from Children." Don't store DMSO in recycled food bottles, even if well-labeled, as this creates a dangerous situation. Avoid storing DMSO in areas accessible to children or pets. DMSO should be in a locked cabinet, on a high shelf, or in another secure location. Don't leave DMSO bottles open or loosely capped, as DMSO absorbs moisture from the air, diluting itself and potentially introducing contaminants.

DMSO Shelf Life: When to Use It and When to Toss It

When stored properly in sealed containers away from light and heat, pharmaceutical-grade DMSO maintains its purity for an extended period. Most manufacturers list expiration dates of two to three years from the manufacturing date, though some high-quality products can remain stable for up to five years under ideal storage conditions. The expiration date on your bottle reflects the manufacturer's guarantee of full potency and purity when you follow their storage instructions exactly.

The key factor affecting shelf life is exposure to air and moisture. DMSO doesn't suddenly become dangerous after its expiration date, but its purity may decrease gradually as it absorbs water from any air exposure. If you're using DMSO past its listed expiration date, understand that the concentration might be lower than what the label states, which affects how you should dilute it for use. For maximum safety and effectiveness, purchase quantities you'll use within the manufacturer's stated shelf life.

When to Throw It Out: 4 Signs Your DMSO Is Contaminated

Fresh pharmaceutical-grade DMSO is clear and colorless. If your DMSO develops a yellow or brown tint, that's a sign of degradation or contamination. Discard it. If you notice particles, cloudiness, or sediment, don't use it. This indicates contamination. If the odor changes significantly (DMSO has a characteristic garlic-like smell, but if it smells chemically different or particularly unpleasant beyond the normal odor, that's concerning). If the bottle has been exposed to contamination (left open, stored improperly, exposed to other chemicals), err on the side of caution and replace it.

Childproofing Your DMSO Storage

If you have children in your home, take extra precautions. Store DMSO in a locked cabinet or on a high shelf completely out of reach. Use childproof caps if available. Never store DMSO in containers that might appeal to children (like old juice bottles or anything with bright colors or familiar labels). Teach older children that this is medicine, not a toy, and explain why they shouldn't touch it. Keep the poison control number readily available. In the United States, that's 1-800-222-1222.

Pets also deserve consideration. Store DMSO where curious pets can't knock it over or access it. If you have a dog or cat that likes to investigate cabinets, make sure your storage location is truly secure.

By following these storage guidelines, you'll maintain your DMSO's quality and safety throughout its shelf life. Proper storage is just as important as buying the right product in the first place. Don't let poor storage practices undermine the care you took in selecting pharmaceutical-grade DMSO.

Chapter Three

Safety First: Your Complete Guide to Risk-Free DMSO Use

Safe use begins long before the first drop of DMSO touches your skin. A little care and preparation go a long way in protecting you from irritation, unexpected reactions, and preventable mistakes. It is important to learn how to patch test correctly, prepare your skin the right way, apply DMSO with confidence, and recognize the difference between normal reactions and warning signs. With these skills in place, DMSO becomes much easier to use safely and comfortably.

The Mandatory Patch Test: Checking for Skin Sensitivity Before Your First Use

Why Patch Testing Is Non-Negotiable

Everyone's skin is different. What works perfectly for one person might cause a severe reaction in another. You cannot predict how your skin will respond without testing. Sensitivity varies not just between people, but even between different areas on your own body. Your inner arm might handle DMSO fine, while your neck reacts badly.

Because of DMSO's draw-through effect, reactions aren't just surface-level. The irritation can go deeper. If you skip the patch test and apply DMSO to your entire knee or shoulder, you might discover hours later that your skin is burning, red, and blistered. Now you have a bigger problem than the pain you were trying to treat.

Complete Patch Test Protocol: Six Essential Steps

Step 1: Choose your test site. The inner forearm is ideal. This area tends to react similarly to other parts of your body and is easy to observe.

Step 2: Clean and dry the test area thoroughly. Wash with fragrance-free soap and water. Rinse completely. Pat dry. Make sure there's no lotion, deodorant, or perfume on the skin.

Step 3: Dilute your DMSO for testing. Start with 50% DMSO diluted with distilled water. Mix equal parts DMSO and distilled water. You only need a teaspoon of each.

Step 4: Apply a small amount. Put a few drops on your inner forearm. Spread it over an area about the size of a quarter.

Step 5: Leave it alone and observe. Don't cover the area. Let it air dry. You need to observe for 24 to 48 hours.

Step 6: Check for reactions at regular intervals. Look at the test site after 30 minutes, 2 hours, 4 hours, the next morning, and after 48 hours. Watch for redness, swelling, itching, burning, blistering, or unusual reactions.

Reading Your Results: What Each Reaction Means

No reaction or very mild redness that fades quickly: You've passed. You can proceed to use DMSO at that concentration or lower.

Mild redness that persists for several hours: You have some sensitivity. Use a lower concentration, like 30%. Limit frequency and avoid sensitive areas.

Moderate reaction with significant redness, itching, or slight swelling: Warning sign. Try a 20% to 30% dilution and test again. If you still react, DMSO might not be right for you.

Severe reaction with intense burning, swelling, blistering, or hives: Stop immediately. Wash the area thoroughly. Apply a cool compress. If the reaction is severe or doesn't improve quickly, seek medical attention.

Some warmth or tingling is normal with DMSO. That's different from burning or pain. Warmth that's tolerable and fades is fine. Burning that intensifies is not.

When Results Aren't Clear: Handling Delayed or Unclear Reactions

If you notice redness the next day, your skin is sensitive to DMSO. Proceed cautiously with lower concentrations. If you're not sure whether redness was from DMSO or something else, repeat the patch test on a different area. This will either confirm sensitivity or show that the first reaction was a false alarm.

If your forearm test went fine, but you want to use DMSO on a sensitive area like your neck, do another patch test there first using a lower concentration of 30% or less. If 50% DMSO caused a mild reaction, test again with 30%. Keep stepping down until you find a level your skin tolerates. Some people can only use 20% to 25% DMSO, and that's fine.

Track your patch test results by noting the date, concentration tested, where you tested it, and what reaction you observed. This helps if you need to talk to a doctor and helps you remember what you tried before.

Skin Prep Essentials: The Critical Steps Before Every Application

Why Skin Prep Is Critical

DMSO doesn't just sit on your skin like most lotions. It penetrates rapidly and deeply, carrying substances with it across the skin barrier. This property is useful in medical settings for delivering medications, but it also means DMSO can deliver contaminants.

Think about what might be on your skin: dirt and bacteria, residue from soap or lotion, perfume, natural oils, cleaning chemicals, pesticides. All of these can potentially be carried into your bloodstream by DMSO. Some substances are harmless in tiny amounts. Others aren't. Proper skin preparation takes just a few minutes and dramatically reduces the risk of introducing unwanted substances into your body.

Five-Step Skin Cleansing Protocol

Step 1: Remove clothing or jewelry from the application area. You need completely unobstructed access to clean skin.

Step 2: Wash with fragrance-free, residue-free soap. Use simple, gentle soap without added moisturizers, fragrances, or antibacterial chemicals. Plain glycerin soap or basic unscented hand soap works well.

Step 3: Rinse thoroughly with clean water. Run water over the area for at least 30 seconds. Make sure you've rinsed away all soap. Soap residue can be carried into your skin by DMSO.

Step 4: Pat the area completely dry with a clean towel. Don't rub vigorously. Make sure the area is completely dry. DMSO will dilute itself if applied to damp skin.

Step 5: Wait a few minutes before applying DMSO. Let your skin return to its normal state after washing.

Never Apply These: Products That Create Dangerous Combinations

Avoid these on or near the application area for several hours before using DMSO:

Lotions and moisturizers contain chemicals, fragrances, and preservatives you don't want in your bloodstream.

Perfumes, colognes, and scented products contain alcohol and fragrance chemicals that can cause irritation when carried through the skin. This includes scented deodorants, body sprays, and hair products.

Sunscreen contains chemical or mineral ingredients that should stay on the surface. If you need sun protection, use clothing or shade. Apply DMSO in the evening after you're done being outside.

Topical medications like pain creams, antibiotic ointments, or steroid creams should not be combined with DMSO unless specifically directed by a doctor. The draw-through effect could intensify these medications unpredictably.

Bug spray and insect repellent contain chemicals like DEET that you don't want delivered into your bloodstream. If you've used bug spray, wash thoroughly and wait several hours before applying DMSO.

Cleaning chemicals require thorough washing before DMSO use. If you've been cleaning with bleach, ammonia, or other household cleaners, wait until the next day to use DMSO.

Quick Pre-Application Checklist

☐ Remove jewelry and clothing from the area

☐ Confirm no lotions, perfumes, or other products applied today

☐ Wash with fragrance-free soap

☐ Rinse thoroughly for at least 30 seconds

☐ Pat completely dry

☐ Wait 2 to 3 minutes

☐ Visually inspect the skin (no cuts, rashes, or irritation)

☐ Ready to apply DMSO

Applying DMSO Correctly: Best Practices and Critical Mistakes to Avoid

Eight Best Practices for Safe Application

1. Use clean, gloved hands or applicators. Wash your hands thoroughly before handling DMSO. Better yet, wear disposable nitrile gloves. If you're using applicators like cotton balls or swabs, use fresh ones from a sealed package.

2. Apply in a well-ventilated area. DMSO has a distinctive odor that can be mildly irritating in enclosed spaces. Open a window or turn on a fan.

3. Use only your recommended dilution. If your patch test showed you tolerate 50% DMSO, don't suddenly jump to 70%. Stick with concentrations you've tested.

4. Apply the right amount for the area. A thin, even layer is sufficient. For a small area like a wrist, a few drops are enough. For a larger area like a knee, you might need a teaspoon. Don't drench the skin.

5. Spread it evenly. Use gentle, smooth motions. Don't rub vigorously. Gentle spreading provides good coverage.

6. Apply to the specific problem area. If your left knee hurts, apply DMSO to your left knee, not the surrounding areas. This minimizes exposure and focuses benefits where needed.

7. Let it air dry for at least 20 minutes. After application, let the DMSO absorb naturally. Don't cover immediately with clothing or bandages.

8. Wash your hands thoroughly after application. Even if you wear gloves, wash your hands to prevent accidental transfer of DMSO.

Seven Critical Mistakes That Compromise Safety

1. Applying to broken, irritated, or infected skin. If you have cuts, scrapes, open wounds, active rashes, sunburn, or any break in the skin barrier, do not apply DMSO. The draw-through effect becomes unpredictable when skin is compromised.

2. Mixing DMSO with unknown or untested substances. Unless you've researched a specific combination thoroughly, don't do it. Stick with proven combinations or use DMSO alone.

3. Covering the area with plastic wrap or occlusive dressings. Occlusive coverings can increase absorption to unsafe levels and trap moisture. Let the area breathe.

4. Applying right before bed if covering the area. While you need to let DMSO air dry before getting dressed, avoid sleeping directly on a freshly treated area. If applying in the evening, do it at least an hour before bed and wear loose clothing.

5. Using more frequently than recommended. If your protocol calls for once-daily application, don't apply it three times a day. More frequent application increases exposure without necessarily increasing benefits and can irritate your skin.

6. Applying to mucous membranes or near the eyes. DMSO should never go on or near your eyes, inside your nose, in your mouth, or on your genital areas. These tissues are much more sensitive. Accidental eye contact requires immediate flushing with water and medical attention if irritation persists.

7. Ignoring early warning signs. If you notice unusual redness, increasing pain, swelling, or unexpected reactions during or after application, stop using DMSO and assess what's happening.

Step-by-Step Application Process

1. Measure the amount of diluted DMSO you need into a small, clean glass or HDPE container.

2. Put on clean gloves or prepare your applicator.

3. Dip your gloved finger, cotton ball, or applicator into the DMSO.

4. Apply to the clean, dry treatment area using gentle, even strokes.

5. Spread in a thin, uniform layer covering the problem area.

6. Set a timer for 20 to 30 minutes.

7. Wash your hands and clean any applicators.

8. After the DMSO has dried, you can cover the area with loose, clean clothing.

Aftercare and Post-Application Hygiene

Dispose of gloves properly. Throw away cotton balls or swabs. Don't reuse applicators. Clean any containers or tools with hot, soapy water. Let them air dry completely.

Monitor the treated area over the next several hours. Some mild warmth or slight redness that fades is normal. Persistent irritation, increasing redness, or discomfort is not normal and suggests you need to adjust your approach.

Recognizing Normal Reactions vs. Warning Signs: When to Seek Medical Help

Normal Side Effects: What to Expect and Why They Happen

Garlic or oyster-like body odor is the most common side effect. DMSO is metabolized into dimethyl sulfide, which has a distinctive smell. This odor can come from your breath and through your pores. It's completely harmless, just socially awkward. The smell typically appears within 15 to 30 minutes and can last for several hours or into the next day.

Mild warmth or tingling at the application site is very common. DMSO creates a warming sensation as it penetrates. This should feel like gentle heat, not burning. Both sensations typically fade within 20 to 30 minutes.

Slight redness at the application site can occur, especially when you first start using DMSO. Mild pinkness that fades within an hour or two is normal. This often decreases as your skin adjusts over multiple applications.

Occasional dryness or mild peeling can happen with regular use. DMSO can have a drying effect on skin. This is usually mild and can be managed by moisturizing several hours after DMSO has fully absorbed.

A taste sensation in your mouth sometimes occurs even though you're applying DMSO to your skin. Some people report tasting garlic or oysters shortly after application. This is the DMSO circulating through your system and is harmless.

Minimizing DMSO's Distinctive Odor: Six Practical Strategies

The garlic odor bothers some people. Here are strategies to minimize it:

1. Apply DMSO in the evening when you're done with social interactions. By morning, the odor is usually less noticeable.

2. Shower several hours after application once it's fully absorbed. This can help reduce residual odor.

3. Drink plenty of water. Staying hydrated helps your body process and eliminate DMSO more efficiently.

4. Use fragrance-free personal care products. Adding perfumes doesn't mask the DMSO smell and can create an unpleasant combination.

5. Wash your clothes promptly if DMSO got on them. The odor can linger in fabric.

6. Be honest with people close to you. Let family or roommates know you're using DMSO.

Most people are understanding when they know it's for pain relief.

Red Flags: Serious Reactions Requiring Immediate Action

Severe burning sensation that intensifies or doesn't fade is not normal. Mild warmth is fine. Actual burning pain is not. If you experience severe burning, immediately wash the area thoroughly with soap and water. Don't apply DMSO again without adjusting your dilution or consulting a healthcare provider.

Blistering or hives indicate an allergic reaction or severe irritation. Stop using DMSO immediately. Wash the area gently. Apply cool compresses if needed. If blistering is extensive or hives spread, seek medical attention.

Significant swelling at the application site is concerning. Mild, temporary puffiness can occur, but obvious swelling that persists or worsens requires stopping DMSO and possibly seeing a doctor.

Shortness of breath, chest tightness, or difficulty breathing could indicate an allergic reaction. Stop using DMSO immediately and seek emergency medical care. These symptoms are rare but require immediate attention.

Persistent headache or nausea after application might indicate sensitivity. Occasional mild headaches can happen when you first start using DMSO, but persistent or severe headaches warrant stopping use.

Skin that stays red, painful, or irritated for more than a few hours suggests the concentration is too strong or your skin is reacting badly. Mild redness that fades is fine. Persistent, intensifying redness with pain is not.

The Truth About "Detox" Reactions: Separating Myth from Reality

Some people talk about "detox reactions" from DMSO, supposedly including temporary fatigue, mild flu-like symptoms, or headaches as DMSO helps the body "release toxins." Be skeptical. While some people experience mild fatigue or headaches when starting DMSO, attributing this to "detoxing" isn't scientifically supported. These symptoms more likely indicate your body is adjusting to a new substance or you're having a mild sensitivity reaction.

If you experience headaches, fatigue, or flu-like symptoms after starting DMSO, reduce your dose, use a lower concentration, or apply it less frequently. These symptoms shouldn't be severe or persistent. If they are, DMSO might not be right for you. Don't push through uncomfortable symptoms thinking you're "detoxing." Pain and discomfort are signals that something is wrong, not signs that healing is happening.

When to Consult a Healthcare Professional

Talk to a doctor if you have a severe reaction or persistent side effects that don't improve with dose reduction. You should also seek medical advice if you notice new or unusual symptoms after starting DMSO, if you're unsure whether a reaction is normal, if you have underlying health conditions or take multiple medications, or if side effects interfere with your daily life. When talking to a healthcare provider, bring information about the product you're using (brand, concentration, purity), how you're using it (dilution, frequency, application sites), and what symptoms you've experienced.

Emergency Response: What to Do for Spills, Eye Contact, and Accidental Ingestion

Immediate Response to Skin Spills: Five Critical Steps

If you spill DMSO on your skin or realize you've applied too much, act quickly.

Step 1: Rinse immediately with copious amounts of cool water. Get to a sink or shower and run cool water over the affected area for at least 10 to 15 minutes. The goal is to dilute and wash away as much DMSO as possible before it fully absorbs.

Step 2: Remove any contaminated clothing. If DMSO gets on your clothes, take them off immediately. DMSO can continue to absorb through fabric.

Step 3: Wash the area with mild soap. After the initial water rinse, gently wash with mild, fragrance-free soap. Rinse thoroughly again.

Step 4: Do not try to neutralize with other chemicals. Don't use vinegar, baking soda, or other household substances. Water and mild soap are all you need.

Step 5: Monitor the area. Watch for redness, irritation, or burning over the next several hours. If symptoms develop or worsen, contact a healthcare provider.

If you spilled DMSO on a surface, clean it up with paper towels, then wash the area with soap and water. Dispose of contaminated paper towels in the trash.

Emergency Eye Exposure Protocol: Act Within Seconds

Eye exposure to DMSO is a serious emergency.

Step 1: Flush the affected eye immediately with clean, lukewarm water. Hold your eye open under gently running water or use an eyewash station. Continue flushing for at least 15 minutes. This is not optional. Fifteen full minutes of continuous flushing.

Step 2: Do not rub the eye. Rubbing can cause more irritation and potentially damage the eye surface.

Step 3: Remove contact lenses if you're wearing them. If you can do this easily during flushing, remove contacts. If they don't come out easily, continue flushing and let medical professionals remove them.

Step 4: Seek medical attention. Even if irritation seems to improve after flushing, see a doctor or go to urgent care. Call ahead and tell them what happened.

Step 5: Bring the DMSO container or product information. Medical professionals will want to know the exact product, concentration, and purity.

Do not use eye drops or any other products unless specifically instructed by a medical professional.

If DMSO Is Swallowed: Emergency Steps to Take Immediately

If someone accidentally swallows DMSO, this is a medical emergency, especially if the amount is more than a few drops.

Step 1: Do not induce vomiting. Do not try to make the person throw up.

Step 2: Call Poison Control immediately. In the United States, the number is 1-800-222-1222. Have the DMSO container with you when you call.

Step 3: Follow Poison Control's instructions exactly. They may tell you to rinse the mouth with water, drink water, or simply monitor. Do exactly what they say.

Step 4: Provide specific information. Be ready to tell Poison Control the concentration of DMSO, how much was ingested, when it happened, and the age and weight of the person.

Step 5: Monitor for symptoms. Watch for nausea, vomiting, abdominal pain, headache, dizziness, or unusual symptoms. Report these to Poison Control.

Step 6: Seek emergency medical care if instructed or if symptoms are severe. If Poison Control tells you to go to the emergency room, go. If the person shows severe symptoms (difficulty breathing, loss of consciousness, severe pain), call 911.

Keep the DMSO container to show medical professionals.

Protecting Children and Pets: Prevention and Emergency Response

If a child or pet gets into your DMSO, treat it as an emergency. For children, follow the same protocols above, depending on how exposure occurred. Call Poison Control for any exposure. Don't assume a small amount is harmless.

For pets, call your veterinarian or an animal poison control hotline immediately. The ASPCA Animal Poison Control Center can be reached at 1-888-426-4435 (a consultation fee may apply). Provide information about the product and the estimated exposure amount. Do not wait to see if symptoms develop. Call for guidance immediately.

Keeping Emergency Information Accessible

Post emergency numbers near where you store DMSO:

- Poison Control: 1-800-222-1222 (US)
- Local emergency: 911 (US)
- Your doctor's office number
- ASPCA Animal Poison Control: 1-888-426-4435 (if you have pets)

Keep the DMSO Safety Data Sheet (SDS) in the same location. Make sure family members or roommates know where the emergency information is and what to do if there's a DMSO accident. Store DMSO securely to prevent accidental exposure. Use locked cabinets if you have children or pets.

A simple emergency reference card might say:

DMSO EMERGENCY ACTIONS

- **Skin Spill**: Rinse 15 min with cool water. Remove clothing. Wash with soap. Monitor.
- **Eye Contact**: Flush 15 min with lukewarm water. Don't rub. Seek medical care.
- **Ingestion**: Don't induce vomiting. Call Poison Control: 1-800-222-1222. Follow instructions.
- **Child/Pet Exposure**: Call Poison Control (child) or vet/ASPCA (pet) immediately. Have product info ready.

Chapter Four

Getting It Right: How Much DMSO to Use, How Strong, and How Often

You've learned what DMSO is, how it works, and what safety precautions to follow. Now comes the practical question that determines whether DMSO helps or harms: how much should you use, how strong should it be, and how often should you apply it? These aren't minor details. The difference between 30% and 90% DMSO can mean the difference between effective relief and painful skin damage. The difference between once-daily and three-times-daily application can determine whether you build tolerance or develop cumulative irritation.

This chapter provides the practical knowledge you need to use DMSO effectively and safely. You'll learn how to calculate dilutions using simple math that doesn't require scientific training, how to choose the right concentration for different body areas and conditions, how to determine optimal application frequency, and why tracking your usage transforms DMSO from hopeful experiment into measurable therapy. These foundational skills apply whether you're treating arthritis in your hands, recovering from a sports injury, or managing chronic pain. Master these basics, and you'll be equipped to adapt DMSO protocols to your changing needs over time.

Understanding DMSO Dilutions: Simple Math for Safe Concentrations

Walk into a health store or browse online DMSO suppliers, and you'll see products labeled 99.9%, 70%, 50%, and various other percentages. Some sources recommend diluting pharmaceutical-grade DMSO yourself. Others suggest using it straight from the bottle. The conflicting advice creates confusion, and confusion leads to mistakes that can cause unnecessary pain and skin damage.

Understanding dilutions isn't complicated once you grasp what the percentages actually mean and why they matter. The math involved is simple arithmetic that anyone can do without special tools or training. More importantly, understanding dilutions gives you control over your treatment. You're not dependent on pre-mixed products that may not match your needs. You can adjust concentrations precisely for different body areas, experiment systematically to find your optimal strength, and save money by purchasing concentrated DMSO and diluting it yourself.

What Percentage Dilutions Actually Mean

When you see "70% DMSO," that means 70% of the liquid is DMSO and 30% is something else, typically distilled water or aloe vera gel. The percentage tells you the ratio of active ingredient to total volume. A 50% solution is half DMSO and half carrier. A 30% solution is 30 parts DMSO to 70 parts carrier.

Pure DMSO is considered 100% or 99.9%, depending on the pharmaceutical grade purity. This undiluted form is occasionally appropriate for very limited applications on thick-skinned areas in experienced users who've built up tolerance gradually. For most purposes and most people, pure DMSO is too strong. It causes unnecessary irritation and offers no additional therapeutic benefit over properly diluted solutions. The goal isn't to use the strongest concentration possible; it's to use the lowest concentration that provides adequate benefit with minimal side effects.

Why does dilution matter for safety? DMSO's effectiveness comes partly from its ability to penetrate skin and carry other substances with it. At high concentrations, this penetration happens too aggressively, overwhelming your skin's protective mechanisms and causing chemical irritation. Think of it like the difference between a gentle rain that waters a garden and a fire hose that erodes the soil. Both deliver water, but one does it in a way the system can handle, while the other causes damage.

The most commonly recommended concentrations fall into three ranges, each with typical applications. Solutions of 25% to 40% work well for sensitive areas like the face, neck, and inner arms, or for people with generally reactive skin. These gentle concentrations minimize irritation risk while still providing anti-inflammatory and pain-relieving effects. Solutions of 50% to 60% represent the standard concentration for most applications on body areas with normal skin thickness, like knees, shoulders, hips, and back. This range offers a good therapeutic effect with a manageable irritation risk for most users. Solutions of 70% to 80% are appropriate only for thick-skinned areas like elbows, the bottoms of feet, or heavily calloused hands, and only after you've established tolerance at lower concentrations. Starting with these strengths, even in thick-skinned areas, invites problems.

Simple Math for Making Your Own Dilutions

Creating dilutions at home requires only basic arithmetic and careful measurement. The core concept is straightforward: decide what total volume you want to make and what percentage you want it to be, then calculate how much DMSO and how much carrier to combine.

The basic formula works like this: multiply your desired percentage (expressed as a decimal) by your total desired volume to get the amount of DMSO needed. The remaining volume is your carrier. If you want to make 10 milliliters of 60% DMSO solution, multiply 0.60 times 10, which equals 6. You need 6 milliliters of DMSO. The remaining 4 milliliters is your carrier, whether distilled water, aloe vera gel, or another appropriate substance.

Let's work through several practical examples covering the most useful dilutions. For a 50% DMSO solution, which is half DMSO and half carrier, the math is particularly simple. To make 20 milliliters total, you need 10 milliliters of DMSO and 10 milliliters of carrier. To make 30 milliliters, use 15 milliliters of each. This 1:1 ratio makes 50% solutions easy to prepare without calculations.

For a 70% DMSO solution, common for treating areas like arthritic knees or athletic injuries on large muscle groups, the calculation requires slightly more attention. To make 20 milliliters of 70% solution, multiply 0.70 times 20 to get 14 milliliters of DMSO. The remaining 6 milliliters is carrier. The ratio is 7:3, which you can remember as roughly "two-thirds DMSO, one-third carrier." To make 30 milliliters at 70%, you'd use 21 milliliters of DMSO and 9 milliliters of carrier.

For a 30% DMSO solution, appropriate for facial applications or very sensitive skin, the ratios reverse. To make 10 milliliters at 30%, multiply 0.30 times 10 to get 3 milliliters of DMSO. Add 7 milliliters of carrier. The ratio is 3:7, or roughly "one-third DMSO, two-thirds carrier." To make 20 milliliters at 30%, use 6 milliliters of DMSO and 14 milliliters of carrier.

These calculations work regardless of whether you're measuring in milliliters, teaspoons, or tablespoons, though milliliters provide the most precision. For reference, one teaspoon equals approximately 5 milliliters, and one tablespoon equals approximately 15 milliliters. If you're making a 50% solution and want enough to fill a small dropper bottle, you might make 30 milliliters using

2 tablespoons of DMSO and 2 tablespoons of carrier. For a 70% solution in the same volume, you'd use roughly 2 tablespoons of DMSO and 1 tablespoon plus 1 teaspoon of carrier.

Quick Reference for Common Ratios

Three ratios cover most DMSO applications, and memorizing them eliminates the need for calculation each time you mix a batch. A 1:1 ratio (equal parts DMSO and carrier) produces 50% concentration. This works perfectly for standard applications on normal skin when you've established tolerance. Mix equal volumes, and you're done. A 7:3 ratio (seven parts DMSO to three parts carrier) produces 70% concentration. This slightly stronger solution suits thicker-skinned areas or users who've found 50% insufficient after adequate trial. A 3:7 ratio (three parts DMSO to seven parts carrier) produces 30% concentration, ideal for sensitive areas or first-time users, being appropriately conservative.

When you see these ratios, remember that they're describing parts of the total volume, not separate measurements added together. The 7:3 ratio means that in every 10 units of solution, 7 units are DMSO and 3 units are carrier. The total is always 10 parts when you add the two numbers in the ratio.

Essential Tools and Techniques for Accurate Measurement

Precision matters when making DMSO dilutions because the difference between 60% and 80% is the difference between effective and irritating. Guessing at measurements or using approximate volumes invites problems. Invest in proper measuring tools, and your dilutions will be consistent, safe, and effective.

Glass measuring cups work well for larger batches, particularly those marked in milliliters rather than just ounces and cups. Look for laboratory-grade or kitchen measuring cups with clear milliliter markings. Avoid plastic measuring cups unless they're specifically HDPE plastic #2, which is DMSO-safe. Regular plastic measuring cups may react with DMSO, leaching chemicals into your solution.

For smaller volumes and maximum precision, oral syringes provide the best measurement tool. These are available at pharmacies without a prescription, typically in 1-milliliter, 3-milliliter, 5-milliliter, and 10-milliliter sizes. They allow you to measure exact amounts, particularly important when making small batches or when working with higher concentrations where a milliliter of difference matters. The wide availability and low cost of oral syringes make them ideal for home DMSO preparation.

Glass containers for mixing and storage are essential, not optional. DMSO reacts with many plastics, metals, and other materials. Glass is completely inert and won't contaminate your solution. Brown or amber glass bottles protect DMSO from light degradation, though clear glass works if you store bottles in a dark location. Make sure containers have tight-fitting caps to prevent evaporation and moisture absorption from the air.

Never use metal utensils or containers when working with DMSO. Metal can react with DMSO, potentially contaminating your solution with metal compounds that DMSO will then carry through your skin. Use glass stirring rods, plastic spatulas from HDPE material, or wooden craft sticks for mixing.

Labeling every batch you make prevents dangerous confusion. Your label should include the concentration (e.g., "60% DMSO"), the carrier used (e.g., "in aloe vera gel"), and the date you mixed it. If you're making multiple dilutions for different body areas or different family members, clear labeling prevents accidentally using 80% formulated for your knee on your face, or using your spouse's batch when you need your own. Use a permanent marker on tape or adhesive labels that won't fall off.

The process of mixing requires care but isn't complicated. Add your carrier to the container first, then add DMSO slowly while stirring gently. DMSO generates heat when mixed with water-based carriers due to an exothermic reaction. This is normal and harmless, but adding DMSO too quickly to water can create surprising warmth. By adding carrier first and DMSO second, you minimize this effect. If using aloe vera gel or oils as carriers, the heat generation is less pronounced. Stir thoroughly for at least 30 seconds to ensure complete mixing, longer if using thick carriers like aloe gel. Allow water-based solutions to cool to room temperature before capping and storing.

Store your prepared dilutions in a cool, dark place away from heat sources and sunlight. DMSO is stable, but extreme temperatures and light can degrade it over time. Label your storage location clearly if others in your household might mistake DMSO solutions for other products. Keep DMSO away from food storage areas to prevent any possibility of contamination or confusion.

Cleanliness throughout the preparation process prevents contamination. Wash your hands thoroughly before handling DMSO or measuring tools. Ensure all containers and utensils are clean and dry before use. If you're diluting from a large stock bottle of pharmaceutical-grade DMSO, avoid contaminating the stock by never pouring it back after you've measured it out. Pour what you need into a clean measuring device, use it, and if you've measured too much, either make a larger batch than planned or discard the excess. The small waste is preferable to contaminating your entire stock bottle.

With these tools and techniques, you can prepare any dilution you need with confidence that it matches your intended concentration. The consistency this precision provides allows you to experiment systematically, knowing that when you try 60% instead of 50%, you're actually testing different concentrations rather than introducing random variation that makes results impossible to interpret.

Choosing Your Starting Strength: Matching Concentration to Body Location and Condition

Knowing how to calculate dilutions solves the technical problem of mixing DMSO correctly. The strategic problem remains: which concentration should you actually use? A 30% solution that works beautifully on your temples might be completely inadequate for your arthritic knee. A 70% solution that provides excellent relief on your shoulder could cause severe irritation on your neck. Getting this decision right from the start prevents the frustrating cycle of trial and error that leaves many people either undertreated or suffering unnecessary skin reactions.

The good news is that you don't need to guess. Decades of clinical use and research have established clear patterns about which concentrations work best for different conditions and body locations. While individual variation exists and you'll need to fine-tune based on your personal response, starting with evidence-based guidelines dramatically increases your chances of finding effective treatment quickly without experiencing preventable problems.

Decision Guidelines for Common Conditions

Different conditions benefit from different starting approaches based on their nature and the typical body locations involved. Thinking through these decision points systematically helps you choose wisely rather than arbitrarily.

For arthritis affecting hands or fingers, start with 40% to 50% DMSO in a moisturizing carrier like aloe vera gel. Hand skin varies in thickness between the back of the hand (thicker, more tolerant) and the spaces between fingers (thinner, more sensitive). The moderate concentration provides anti-inflammatory effects while accounting for this variation. Apply once daily initially, typically in the evening, so any mild irritation doesn't interfere with daytime activities requiring hand dexterity. If you tolerate 50% well for two weeks with good but incomplete relief, consider increasing to 60%. If 40% causes any stinging or prolonged redness, reduce to 30% before trying again.

For arthritis in knees, hips, or shoulders, begin with 50% to 60% DMSO. These large joints have thicker overlying skin and substantial underlying tissue requiring adequate DMSO penetration to reach the affected joint structures. Start with a once-daily application, preferably before physical activity or therapy, when pain reduction helps you move more effectively. The skin over these joints can typically tolerate 60% without problems in most users. If pain relief is inadequate after two weeks at 60% with consistent daily application, you can trial 70%, but this increase should come with careful monitoring for any skin changes.

For acute injuries like sprains, strains, or impact injuries causing swelling and bruising, use 60% DMSO for the first few days when inflammation is most severe. The goal during acute injury treatment is aggressive anti-inflammatory action to minimize tissue damage and speed recovery. Apply two to three times daily for the first 48 to 72 hours, then reduce frequency as acute inflammation subsides. If the injury involves an area with thinner skin, like the inner arm or ankle, start at 50% even during the acute phase.

For tension headaches or migraines where you're applying DMSO to the neck, temples, or scalp, always start at 25% to 30%, regardless of how well you tolerate higher concentrations elsewhere on your body. The face, neck, and scalp have thin, highly sensitive skin with a rich blood supply. Higher concentrations risk not just local irritation but also systemic effects from rapid absorption. Use the minimal amount needed, typically just a few drops, and apply no more than once per headache episode. Never use DMSO preventively multiple times daily for headache conditions, as this creates unnecessary cumulative exposure in sensitive areas.

When to increase concentration depends on two factors working together: you've tolerated your current concentration well for at least one to two weeks without skin irritation, and you're experiencing incomplete symptom relief despite consistent application. If either factor is missing, don't increase. Good tolerance without adequate relief might mean you need a different treatment entirely, rather than stronger DMSO. Adequate relief, even partial, at your current concentration suggests you've found your effective dose, and increasing serves no purpose.

When to decrease concentration is simpler: any time you experience stinging that lasts more than 30 minutes, redness that persists for more than two hours after application, skin dryness or flaking, or any other adverse skin reaction. Decrease by at least 10% to 15% and allow your skin to fully recover before trying again. If problems persist even at lower concentrations, DMSO might not be appropriate for that particular body area, or you might need a different carrier that's less irritating for your skin type.

Why Body Location Determines Appropriate Strength

Skin thickness varies dramatically across your body, creating a roughly ten-fold difference in tolerance between the thickest and thinnest areas. This variation isn't just about comfort during application; it affects how quickly DMSO absorbs, how deeply it penetrates, and how likely it is to cause both local irritation and systemic effects.

The face, neck, and inner arms represent your most sensitive areas. Skin here is thin, has minimal underlying fat padding, contains high concentrations of nerve endings, and sits close to major blood vessels. These factors combine to create rapid absorption and heightened sensitivity to irritation. For facial applications like treating sinus inflammation, temporal headaches, or TMJ issues, never exceed 40% concentration and typically start at 25% to 30%. For neck applications addressing tension or cervical spine issues, use 30% to 40% maximum. Inner arms, sometimes treated for conditions like lymphedema or localized pain, should also stay in the 30% to 40% range.

Standard body areas, including knees, shoulders, elbows, hips, thighs, calves, and the back, can handle 50% to 70% DMSO safely in most users. These areas have thicker skin, more substantial underlying tissue, and can benefit from stronger concentrations that penetrate deeply enough to reach affected joints, muscles, and connective tissues. Starting at 50% for these locations represents a reasonable balance between effectiveness and safety. Users who tolerate 50% well and need stronger effects can progress to 60% or even 70% after establishing tolerance.

Thick-skinned areas like the soles of feet, heavily calloused hands, or the thick skin over elbows can theoretically tolerate 70% to 80% DMSO, but even these areas benefit from starting more conservatively. Just because skin can tolerate high concentrations doesn't mean high concentrations provide better results. Many users find that 60% on thick-skinned areas provides the same therapeutic benefit as 80% without the risk of cumulative irritation from repeated applications. The exception might be conditions like plantar fasciitis, where the thick plantar skin seems to benefit from higher concentrations to achieve adequate penetration.

The rationale behind these location-based recommendations comes down to creating therapeutic DMSO concentrations in the target tissue without overwhelming the skin's protective capacity. Thin skin over sensitive areas reaches therapeutic tissue concentrations with lower DMSO percentages because there's less barrier to penetration. Thick skin over large joints requires higher percentages to achieve the same tissue concentrations because DMSO must penetrate through a more resistant barrier and travel through more tissue to reach the inflamed joint.

Starting Points and Safe Progression

First-time DMSO users face a choice: start very conservatively to minimize any risk of problems, or start at moderate concentrations likely to provide therapeutic benefit quickly. The wise middle path involves starting at 30% to 50%, depending on the body location you're treating, which provides a reasonable likelihood of benefit while minimizing serious irritation risk.

If you're treating a sensitive area like your face, neck, or inner arms, begin at 30% even as a first-time user. If you're treating standard areas like knees, shoulders, or back, starting at 50% is reasonable. If you're unusually cautious or have a history of sensitive skin or allergic reactions to topical products, starting at 40% for standard areas adds an extra margin of safety. There's no shame in being conservative. You can always increase concentration, but you can't undo skin damage from starting too aggressively.

Gradual concentration increases should follow the 10% to 15% increment rule with one to two weeks between increases. If you start at 40% and tolerate it well but want to try stronger, move to 50% after one to two weeks. After another one to two weeks at 50%, if you're still tolerating it well, you can try 60%. This stepwise approach allows your skin to adapt to increasing concentrations while giving you clear feedback about your tolerance at each level.

The timeline matters as much as the increment size. Jumping from 40% to 50% after only three days doesn't give your skin adequate time to show delayed reactions that might develop with repeated applications. Some irritation appears only after several days of use at a given concentration. Waiting one to two weeks before increasing ensures you're seeing your true tolerance rather than just your initial reaction.

Maximum safe concentrations vary by body area, but general guidelines help prevent overreach. For facial and neck applications, 40% represents a reasonable upper limit for most users. Some people tolerate 50% on the neck, but there's rarely any justification for going higher on these sensitive areas. For standard body areas, 70% is the practical upper limit. A very few users with thick skin and high tolerance might go to 80%, but this should be reserved for specific situations like treating plantar fasciitis, where the extremely thick plantar skin warrants it. For most conditions on most body areas, if 70% isn't providing adequate relief, the problem isn't insufficient concentration. You either need a different treatment, you're not applying frequently enough, or DMSO isn't the right intervention for your particular condition.

Common Mistakes in Choosing Concentrations

Even with clear guidelines, certain mistakes appear repeatedly among DMSO users. Recognizing these patterns helps you avoid them.

Overestimating skin tolerance based on irrelevant factors leads many people astray. Someone might think, "I work construction, I have tough skin, I can handle 80% right from the start." Physical toughness, pain tolerance, and even having calloused skin from manual labor don't predict DMSO tolerance. The chemical irritation from concentrated DMSO is fundamentally different from mechanical stress. Similarly, believing "I need strong treatment for severe pain" doesn't justify starting at maximum concentrations. Pain severity doesn't determine optimal DMSO concentration. Start conservatively regardless of how tough you think you are or how severe your condition feels.

Skipping gradual progression steps out of impatience creates predictable problems. Jumping from 40% to 80% because you're eager for faster relief bypasses the skin adaptation that makes higher concentrations tolerable. Your skin needs time to adjust to DMSO's effects at each concentration level. The slight extra benefit you might get from skipping steps gets overwhelmed by the irritation you cause, often setting you back further than if you'd progressed patiently. Stick to 10% to 15% increases spaced one to two weeks apart. This isn't excessive caution; it's what actually works.

Using the same concentration everywhere on your body is remarkably common and remarkably problematic. The 70% solution that works perfectly on your knee will likely cause significant irritation on your neck, and potentially severe problems on your face. Different body areas require different concentrations. This means you might need to prepare multiple dilutions if you're treating multiple body areas. Keep them clearly labeled and use the right one for each location.

Not patch-testing new concentrations before full application invites unnecessary problems. When you increase from 50% to 60%, test the new concentration on a small area first, about the size of a quarter. Wait 24 to 48 hours. If no irritation develops, proceed with full-area application. This simple step prevents you from covering a large area with a concentration that proves too strong, which would require waiting for widespread irritation to heal before you could try again at a lower strength.

Ignoring early warning signs because you don't want to admit the concentration is too strong delays necessary adjustments and worsens outcomes. Mild stinging that lasts an hour, redness that persists for several hours, or slight dryness developing after a few days are your body's early feedback that you need to adjust. Pushing through these signals, hoping they'll resolve on their own, usually leads to more severe irritation that forces a complete break from DMSO rather than a simple concentration reduction. Early adjustment prevents serious problems. The moment you notice concerning symptoms, reduce your concentration by 10% to 15% and reassess. Catching problems early keeps them manageable.

How Often to Apply: Frequency Guidelines and the Importance of Rest Periods

You've learned how to make the right concentration and match it to the appropriate body area. The next question follows naturally: how often should you actually apply it? This seemingly simple question has a complex answer because optimal frequency depends on multiple factors, including what you're treating, how your skin responds, and how long you've been using DMSO. Apply too infrequently, and you undertreat your condition, leaving pain and inflammation inadequately controlled. Apply too frequently, and you risk cumulative skin irritation, diminishing returns, or potentially developing tolerance where DMSO becomes less effective over time.

The good news is that clear patterns have emerged from decades of clinical use and research. While you'll need to personalize based on your response, starting with evidence-based frequency guidelines prevents the common mistakes that undermine treatment effectiveness or cause unnecessary problems.

Starting Frequency and Building Tolerance

The safest starting point for nearly everyone treating nearly any condition is once-daily application. This conservative frequency allows you to assess how your skin tolerates DMSO at your chosen concentration without the compounding effects of multiple daily applications. You get meaningful therapeutic benefit from once-daily use while minimizing the risk of cumulative irritation that can develop when skin doesn't get adequate recovery time between applications.

Apply at a consistent time each day to establish a routine and make tracking easier. Many people prefer evening application because any mild irritation or the characteristic garlic breath occurs during sleep rather than affecting work or social situations. Others prefer morning application before physical therapy or exercise when DMSO's pain-relieving effects support therapeutic movement. Either timing works; consistency matters more than the specific hour you choose.

Continue once-daily application for at least one to two weeks before considering any increase in frequency. This waiting period serves several purposes. It allows you to assess whether once-daily use provides adequate symptom relief, which it often does for many chronic conditions. It gives your skin time to show delayed reactions that might not appear after just a few applications. And it establishes a baseline against which you can measure whether increased frequency provides additional benefit or just additional irritation.

If once-daily application provides incomplete relief after two weeks of consistent use and your skin tolerates it well with no significant irritation, you can add a second application, typically spacing it roughly 12 hours from the first. Morning and evening applications create this spacing naturally. The second application should use the same concentration that worked well once daily unless you have specific reasons to adjust.

Building to three times daily represents the upper limit of reasonable frequency for most conditions and should be approached cautiously. The only situations typically warranting three-times-daily application are acute injuries during the first few days when inflammation is most severe, or severe chronic pain that inadequately responds to twice-daily dosing. Even when using DMSO three times daily, this frequency should be time-limited, typically no more than five to seven consecutive days before reducing to twice daily, then once daily as the acute phase resolves.

The maximum consecutive days before implementing rest periods varies based on how frequently you're applying DMSO. Once-daily application can continue for weeks to months in many users without requiring scheduled breaks, though watching for any signs of cumulative skin irritation remains important. Twice-daily application should include planned breaks every three to four weeks, typically taking two to three days completely off DMSO to allow the skin to fully recover. Three-times-daily application, when used at all, should be limited to five to seven days maximum before reducing frequency or taking a break.

How DMSO Absorbs and Works in Your Body

Understanding DMSO's timeline in your body helps explain why certain frequency patterns work better than others and why more frequent application doesn't always mean better results.

DMSO, applied topically, penetrates the skin rapidly, with peak tissue concentrations occurring within one to two hours after application. This quick absorption means the bulk of DMSO's delivery into affected tissue happens relatively fast. By two hours post-application, most of the DMSO that's going to penetrate has already done so. This rapid uptake is one reason DMSO works more quickly than many other topical treatments that require hours to penetrate adequately.

The therapeutic effects of a single DMSO application, however, last considerably longer than the absorption period. Anti-inflammatory and analgesic effects typically persist for 12 to 24 hours after a single application, varying based on the condition being treated, the concentration used, and individual factors. This extended duration of action explains why once-daily or twice-daily application works for most conditions rather than requiring continuous reapplication.

Spacing applications matters because skin needs recovery time between DMSO exposures. While DMSO absorbs quickly, the mild chemical irritation it causes takes longer to resolve. Applying DMSO again before the skin has recovered from the previous application creates cumulative irritation that builds over days or weeks. This is why twice-daily applications spaced 12 hours apart work better than two applications separated by just six hours. The longer interval allows the skin more recovery time between exposures.

The relationship between absorption timing and therapeutic duration also explains why applying DMSO more than three times daily rarely provides additional benefit. Since therapeutic effects last 12 to 24 hours and peak tissue concentration occurs within one to two hours, frequent reapplication doesn't increase the therapeutic effect proportionally. You're just adding more cumulative skin exposure without meaningful additional benefit. Finding the minimum frequency that provides adequate symptom control, rather than maximizing frequency hoping for maximal effect, represents the wiser approach.

Tailoring Frequency to Specific Conditions

Different conditions require different frequency strategies based on their nature, severity, and expected healing timeline.

Acute injuries, including sprains, strains, impact injuries, and post-surgical swelling, benefit from aggressive initial treatment with subsequent tapering. Apply DMSO three times daily during the first three to five days when acute inflammation is most severe and aggressive anti-inflammatory action provides maximum benefit. Space applications roughly eight hours apart if possible, typically morning, mid-afternoon, and evening. After three to five days, as acute inflammation subsides, reduce to twice-daily application for another week. Then taper to once-daily application for an additional one to two weeks as healing continues. This tapering schedule matches DMSO frequency to the injury's changing inflammatory status rather than maintaining high frequency longer than necessary.

Chronic arthritis and ongoing joint pain typically respond well to once or twice-daily application without the aggressive initial loading used for acute injuries. Start with a once-daily application for two weeks. If pain relief is adequate, continue at this frequency. If relief is incomplete, increase to twice daily. Even with chronic conditions requiring ongoing DMSO use, implement periodic breaks every three to four weeks. Take two to three full days off DMSO, then resume your regular schedule. These breaks prevent cumulative skin irritation and may prevent the development of tolerance where DMSO becomes less effective over time.

Headaches and migraines require a completely different approach than musculoskeletal conditions. Apply DMSO only during acute headache episodes, not as a preventive measure, multiple times daily. Use it once at headache onset, applying to the neck, temples, or other appropriate areas. If the headache doesn't improve adequately within two to four hours, you can apply a second time, but avoid repeated applications throughout the day. Never use DMSO multiple times daily, every day, as headache prevention. This creates unnecessary exposure in sensitive areas like the face and neck without proven preventive benefit.

Implementing "off weeks" becomes necessary when you've been using DMSO twice daily for extended periods. After three to four weeks of twice-daily application, take a full week off or reduce to once every other day for a week. This break serves multiple purposes. It allows your skin extended recovery time, reducing the risk of cumulative irritation. It resets your baseline so you can assess your true symptom level without DMSO's influence, helping you determine whether continued treatment remains necessary. And it may prevent tolerance development, though the evidence for DMSO tolerance in humans is limited. Some users find that periodic breaks actually enhance DMSO's effectiveness when they resume, possibly due to skin recovering its full absorption capacity or inflammatory processes resetting.

Discovering Your Personal Optimal Routine

The frequency guidelines provided represent evidence-based starting points, but your optimal routine emerges through careful observation of two key factors working together.

Skin tolerance tells you the maximum frequency you can sustain safely. If you notice increasing redness, persistent stinging, dryness, or other irritation developing over days or weeks of use, your frequency exceeds your skin's tolerance at that concentration. Reduce frequency by dropping one application per day, or implement more frequent break days. If skin problems develop even at once-daily application, the issue might be concentration rather than frequency, warranting dilution to a lower percentage before adjusting frequency.

Symptom relief tells you the minimum frequency you need for adequate treatment. If once-daily application controls your pain and inflammation adequately, there's no reason to increase frequency just because guidelines allow twice daily. Use the minimum frequency that achieves your functional goals. If once-daily application provides only partial relief and twice-daily offers substantially better symptom control without causing skin problems, twice daily becomes your optimal frequency.

The intersection of these factors defines your ideal routine. You want the frequency that provides adequate symptom control without causing progressive skin irritation. This might be once daily, twice daily, or even every other day, depending on your condition, skin sensitivity, and treatment goals. There's no universal answer, which is why systematic tracking of both your symptoms and skin response becomes invaluable for finding your personal optimal frequency.

Why Tracking Matters: Building a Simple System to Optimize Your Results

You now understand how to dilute DMSO correctly, choose appropriate concentrations for different body areas, and determine optimal application frequency. These skills give you the technical foundation for effective DMSO use. But there's one more practice that separates people who get mediocre results from those who optimize DMSO to its full potential: systematic tracking of what you're doing and how your body responds.

Tracking feels tedious. It adds steps to your routine. It requires consistency when you're already managing pain or dealing with injury. But the return on this small investment is enormous. Tracking transforms DMSO from a hopeful experiment into measurable therapy where you know what works, can replicate successes, and can identify problems before they become serious. If you take away only one practice from this chapter beyond safe application itself, make it tracking.

Why Your Memory Isn't Good Enough

Human memory excels at many things, but accurately tracking subtle patterns over weeks or months isn't among them. Your brain prioritizes recent experiences, emotionally charged events, and simplified narratives over the granular detail needed to optimize a therapeutic protocol. This creates predictable distortions that undermine your ability to use DMSO effectively.

Consider what happens without tracking. You start using DMSO for knee pain. Some days your knee feels better, some days worse. After three weeks, you try to assess whether DMSO is actually helping. Your brain recalls the really good days and the really bad days, but fuzzes over the average days that make up most of your experience. You might conclude "DMSO helps sometimes but not consistently" when the actual data, if you'd tracked it, would show that your average pain decreased from seven out of ten to four out of ten, a clinically significant improvement that got obscured by focusing on the variability.

Tracking reveals patterns that memory simply cannot detect. Without tracking, you might think DMSO's effectiveness varies randomly. With tracking, you discover that 60% concentration applied in the morning provides six to seven hours of meaningful relief, while 50% applied at bedtime provides only three to four hours but causes less morning stiffness. This specificity allows you to optimize your protocol: use 60% in the morning on active days when you need sustained relief, and 50% at night on rest days when minimizing morning stiffness matters more.

Similarly, without tracking, you might conclude that DMSO inevitably irritates your skin after a week or so of use. With tracking, you discover the irritation appears specifically on days eight to nine of consecutive use, and only when you've applied twice daily for three consecutive days prior to the irritation appearing. Armed with this pattern, you can preemptively schedule 48-hour breaks on day seven, preventing irritation entirely rather than just reacting to it after it develops.

Without tracking, you might feel that DMSO helped initially but doesn't work as well anymore, leading you to abandon what could have been effective long-term treatment. With tracking, you see that your pain relief ratings dropped from eight out of ten improvement to five out of ten over three weeks, but your application frequency also unconsciously decreased from daily to three to four times weekly during that same period. The diminished results aren't tolerance or DMSO becoming less effective. They're inconsistent use. Restoring daily application restores full benefits, which you'd never realize without data showing the correlation.

These aren't theoretical examples. They represent the most common patterns users discover when they begin tracking systematically. Your specific patterns will differ based on your condition, your skin sensitivity, and your individual response to DMSO, but they're equally discoverable and equally valuable for optimizing your treatment.

Beyond helping you optimize your personal protocol, tracking creates the foundation for productive communication with healthcare providers. When you can present objective data showing what you've tried, what concentrations and frequencies you've used, and what results you've achieved, you transform conversations with doctors, physical therapists, and other providers from vague discussions into data-driven problem-solving. Chapter 8 covers in detail how to use your tracking data for provider communication, but the foundation starts here with building the habit of consistent documentation.

Simple Tools to Get Started

Effective tracking doesn't require elaborate systems, expensive apps, or time-consuming documentation. The best tracking method is the one you'll actually use consistently. For most people, this means starting simple and building complexity only if and when it adds value.

The notebook method works beautifully for many users. Keep a small notebook or journal dedicated to DMSO tracking near your DMSO supplies. Each entry needs only basic information: today's date, the concentration you used, where you applied it, your pain or symptom level before application, rated zero to ten, and your pain or symptom level two to four hours after application, also rated zero to ten. This takes perhaps 60 to 90 seconds to record. At the end of the week, you have seven entries showing patterns in your response. At the end of a month, you have enough data to make informed decisions about adjusting your protocol.

The phone notes app approach uses technology that most people already carry with them constantly. Create a note titled "DMSO Tracking" and add entries using the same basic format as the notebook method. The advantage is that your phone is always with you, making it easy to record entries even when away from home. The disadvantage is that phones have distractions, and it's easy to open your notes app intending to track and instead check messages, social media, or email. If you're disciplined with your phone, this method works well. If you're easily distracted, the physical notebook might serve you better.

Regardless of format, focus initially on three essential data points that provide maximum value for minimum effort. Did you apply DMSO today? What was your pain level before the application? What was your pain level after application? These three questions answered consistently give you the core information needed to assess whether DMSO is helping, whether your current concentration and frequency are optimal, and whether you're experiencing cumulative benefits or diminishing returns over time.

Don't overcomplicate your tracking initially. Resist the temptation to track fifteen variables from day one. You might want to record the carrier you used, the exact time of application, the outdoor temperature, what you ate that day, how much you slept, your stress level, and half a dozen other factors. This level of detail becomes overwhelming quickly, leading most people to abandon tracking entirely within a week. Start with the three essential data points. Track these consistently for two weeks. If you find you want more detail to answer specific questions that emerge, add one or two additional variables. Build gradually rather than starting with complexity that proves unsustainable.

Making Tracking a Consistent Habit

Understanding the value of tracking and knowing what to track solves the intellectual problem. Actually tracking consistently day after day solves the behavioral problem, which for most people is the harder challenge. Habit formation research offers clear guidance on making tracking stick.

Physical proximity creates the strongest habit trigger. Keep your tracking log, whether notebook or dedicated phone, right next to your DMSO supplies. When you reach for your DMSO, you see your tracking tool. This visual cue reminds you to record your entry before application, and again two to four hours later when you rate your pain relief. Many users find it helpful to create a small DMSO station in a drawer or shelf containing their DMSO, carrier agents, applicators, and tracking log all in one place. This bundling makes the entire routine, including tracking, feel like a single unified practice rather than separate steps requiring separate decisions.

Set phone reminders for the first two weeks while the tracking habit is forming. Create a daily alarm for your typical application time with a label like "Apply DMSO and Log Entry." Set a second alarm for two to four hours later, labeled "Rate Pain Relief." These reminders feel excessive and might seem annoying, but they're temporary training wheels, not permanent fixtures. After 10 to 14 days of consistent tracking, the habit typically becomes automatic, and the reminders become unnecessary. You can then turn them off, having successfully established the pattern.

Start minimal and expand gradually rather than attempting comprehensive tracking from day one. Your first week, track only the three essential data points: did you apply, pain before, pain after. Nothing else. This minimal approach feels manageable and builds the core habit. During your second week, continue tracking those three points while considering whether adding one or two more variables would help answer specific questions you have. Perhaps you want to track which concentration you used each day, or which carrier, or the time of day you applied. Add one or two variables maximum. Build gradually over weeks, adding complexity only when the basic habit is solid and when additional data would provide genuine value rather than just feeling more thorough.

Weekly review creates the feedback loop that makes tracking meaningful rather than just data collection. Choose the same day each week, perhaps Sunday evening or Monday morning, and spend five minutes reviewing your entries from the past seven days. Calculate your average pain level for the week. Note your best day and worst day. Look for any patterns in what correlates with better or worse outcomes. Decide whether any protocol adjustments seem warranted based on what you're seeing. This weekly review closes the loop, transforming raw data into actionable insights that actually improve your DMSO use.

Comprehensive Templates and Advanced Tracking

The simple tracking approach outlined here provides everything most DMSO users need to optimize their treatment and communicate effectively with healthcare providers. For users who want more detailed tracking or who are managing complex conditions requiring sophisticated documentation, comprehensive templates can be found in the Bonus section at the end of this book.

The daily DMSO application log in Bonus section includes fields for detailed information beyond the basic three data points, allowing you to track variables like skin reaction ratings, functional capacity measures, medication use for breakthrough pain, and notes about unusual factors that might affect your response. The weekly summary worksheet provides structure for your weekly reviews, prompting you to calculate averages, identify trends, and plan protocol adjustments systematically. Condition-specific tracking sheets tailored to arthritis, injury recovery, chronic pain, and other common DMSO applications include relevant measures for each condition type.

You don't need these detailed templates to begin tracking effectively. The simple approach of notebook or phone notes with three essential data points works well for most users. But when you're ready to optimize further or when you need more sophisticated documentation for provider communication, these templates are available. Chapter 8: Preparing for Success: What to Bring to Medical Appointments covers in detail how to transform your tracking data into presentations for healthcare providers, building on the foundation you're establishing now with basic, consistent documentation.

The goal isn't perfect tracking. The goal is consistent tracking that generates the insights you need to make DMSO work optimally for your situation. Start simple, stay consistent, and let the data guide your way forward.

Make a Difference with Your Review

Unlock the Power of Generosity

"Kind words can be short and easy to speak, but their echoes are truly endless." – Mother Teresa

People who give without expecting anything in return often feel happier and more fulfilled. So if we have a chance to do something good together, I want to take it.

Let me ask you something...

Would you help someone you have never met, even if no one ever knew you did it?

That person is someone just like you. Someone dealing with pain, inflammation, or discomfort, and looking for simple, natural ways to feel better.

The mission of this book is to make DMSO safe, simple, and easy to understand for everyone. The only way to reach more people is with your help.

Most readers choose a book based on reviews. So here is my small request:

Please leave a quick review for this book.

It takes less than 60 seconds, but it could help...

...one more person find relief
...one more person feel hope
...one more person move more freely

Simply scan the QR code or click the link below to leave your review:

https://www.amazon.com/review/review-your-purchases/?asin=B0GWWLW4JM

If you are willing to help someone you may never meet, you are my kind of person.

Thank you for being here. I am excited to keep helping you in the chapters ahead.

Your biggest fan,
Amelia Hartwell

P.S. If this book helped you, consider sharing it with someone who could benefit too.

Chapter Five

From Arthritis to Sports Injuries: Custom DMSO Protocols for Common Conditions

You've mastered the fundamentals of DMSO safety, quality selection, dilution, and dosing. Now comes the practical application: how do you actually use DMSO for the specific conditions that brought you to this book? Arthritis in your hands requires a different approach than a pulled hamstring. Chronic tendonitis demands protocols distinct from acute injury treatment. This chapter provides targeted guidance for the most common DMSO applications, with clear protocols for each condition, decision trees to guide your choices, and troubleshooting advice when standard approaches need adjustment.

DMSO for Arthritis Relief: Protocols for Hands, Knees, and Hips

Arthritis pain varies dramatically by joint location. Your hands face different mechanical stresses than your knees, and your hips endure loads your fingers never experience. Effective DMSO protocols recognize these differences and tailor concentration, application method, and frequency accordingly.

Site-Specific Protocols for Each Joint

Hand and finger arthritis: Start with 40% DMSO in aloe vera gel. Hand skin is thin with high nerve density, making lower concentrations essential. After one week of good tolerance, increase to 50% if needed. Hand applications should rarely exceed 60% DMSO.

Use a cotton swab or clean fingertip to apply a thin layer to affected joints, focusing on the joint itself rather than covering the entire finger. For knuckles, apply to the top surface where skin is thicker, avoiding sensitive palm-side joints when possible.

Apply once daily in the evening, allowing 20 to 30 minutes before washing hands or using hand cream. Evening application minimizes disruption and allows maximum overnight absorption. If increasing to twice daily, add a morning application, but wait 30 to 40 minutes before hand washing. Use 2 to 4 drops per affected joint. The total application should not exceed 1 to 2 milliliters to avoid excessive systemic absorption.

Knee arthritis: The knee's thicker skin, larger surface area, and limited nerve density allow stronger concentrations. Start with 60% DMSO in aloe vera gel. After one week of good tolerance, increase to 70% if additional relief is needed.

Apply with clean hands or a cotton pad to the entire front knee, including above and below the kneecap. Cover the inner and outer aspects of the knee for comprehensive joint capsule coverage.

Apply once or twice daily. Morning application reduces stiffness before daily activities. Evening application addresses accumulated pain from the day's use. Space applications at least 12 hours apart. Use 2 to 3 milliliters per knee (about half a teaspoon). This provides adequate coverage without excess.

Hip arthritis: The hip joint sits deep beneath muscle and tissue. DMSO must penetrate multiple layers to reach the affected joint. Start with 60% DMSO in aloe vera gel or coconut oil. The hip's deep location warrants higher concentrations from the outset. Increase to 70% after one week if well-tolerated and relief is insufficient.

Apply to the front hip crease, outer thigh area, and buttock where hip pain often occurs. Use firm but gentle circular massage during application to enhance penetration. Apply once or twice daily. Use 3 to 5 milliliters per hip distributed across multiple application areas.

Protocol Selection Flowchart

For hands:

- First-time user? Start with 40% in aloe vera

- Good tolerance after one week, but insufficient relief? Increase to 50%
- Skin becomes dry or irritated? Switch to coconut oil carrier or add moisturizer 30 minutes after application
- Knuckles remain swollen despite treatment? Increase frequency to twice daily before increasing concentration

For knees:

- First-time user? Start with 60% in aloe vera
- Experienced user? Start with 60% to 70%
- Good tolerance but insufficient relief after one week? Increase to 70%
- Morning stiffness: primary concern? Apply morning only
- All-day pain? Apply twice daily, morning and evening

For hips:

- Deep, aching pain? Start with 60% in coconut oil for enhanced penetration
- Sharp, surface pain? Start with 60% in aloe vera
- No relief after three weeks at 60% twice daily? Increase to 70%
- Good relief, but skin irritated? Reduce frequency to once daily or take a two-day break weekly

Integrating DMSO with Joint-Supportive Practices

DMSO works best as part of a comprehensive joint health strategy. Apply DMSO 20 to 30 minutes before gentle range-of-motion exercises or physical therapy. The pain relief window creates optimal conditions for therapeutic movement. Never use DMSO to mask pain during high-impact activities. This risks overuse injury.

Alternate DMSO with heat or cold. Apply cold packs for 15 to 20 minutes to reduce acute inflammation, wait 30 minutes, then apply DMSO. Or apply DMSO first, wait 30 to 40 minutes for absorption, then use heat therapy to enhance circulation.

After applying DMSO, use slow, circular motions around the joint to encourage absorption and promote synovial fluid movement.

Troubleshooting Arthritis-Specific Issues

Knuckle swelling versus deep joint pain: If swelling primarily affects knuckles, use 40% DMSO twice daily and consider compression gloves one hour after application. For deep, aching pain without visible swelling, increase to 50% to 60% DMSO and combine with heat therapy. For both swelling and deep pain, start with the swelling protocol, then address deep pain with a higher concentration once swelling reduces.

Timing decisions: Severe morning stiffness? Prioritize evening application since overnight action reduces wake-up stiffness. Pain worsens throughout the day? Prioritize morning application to preempt activity-related inflammation. Both issues? Implement twice-daily protocol with a lower concentration (50% to 60%) to maintain tolerance.

When to pause or consult: Stop DMSO immediately if the joint becomes red, hot, or more swollen after two to four days. This suggests possible infection or inflammatory flare requiring medical evaluation. If pain increases significantly despite regular use, pause for 48 hours. If pain remains elevated, consult a provider for potential underlying progression. If skin develops a persistent rash, scaling, or cracking, stop DMSO and allow five to seven days of recovery before restarting at 50% lower concentration with a different carrier. If you see no improvement after two weeks of consistent use, DMSO may not be effective for your arthritis type. Discuss alternatives with your healthcare provider.

Easing Muscle Aches and Sports Injuries: Step-by-Step Applications

Muscle injuries and sports-related pain respond exceptionally well to DMSO when protocols match the injury timeline and location. Whether dealing with an acute hamstring pull or chronic shoulder tension, the right DMSO approach can dramatically accelerate recovery and restore function.

Acute Versus Chronic Muscle Pain Protocols

Acute injury (first 48 to 72 hours): Begin DMSO as soon as possible after injury, ideally within the first few hours. An earlier application often means faster resolution.

Start with 60% DMSO in aloe vera gel for most muscle injuries. New DMSO users should start at 50% even for acute injuries. Apply three times daily for the first 48 hours, spacing applications six to eight hours apart. This aggressive early frequency capitalizes on DMSO's ability to reduce swelling and pain when tissue damage is fresh.

Apply generously to the entire injured area plus two to three inches beyond the pain zone. Muscle injuries often involve surrounding tissue. Follow modified RICE protocol: Rest, Ice before DMSO (15 minutes), wait 15 minutes, apply DMSO, wait 30 minutes for absorption, then apply compression wrap if appropriate, and Elevation.

Subacute phase (days 4 through 14): Continue with 60% DMSO or reduce to 50% if skin irritation develops. Reduce frequency to twice daily, morning and evening. Begin gentle range-of-motion exercises 30 to 45 minutes after DMSO application. The pain relief window allows therapeutic movement without compensation patterns.

Delayed onset muscle soreness (DOMS): Use 50% DMSO in aloe vera or coconut oil. DOMS involves microtrauma and inflammation but not severe tissue damage. Apply once daily, preferably in the evening. Cover the entire sore muscle group generously. Use for two to five days maximum. If soreness persists beyond four days, you're likely dealing with an actual strain.

Chronic muscle pain: Start with 50% DMSO and adjust based on response. Some chronic conditions respond better to 60% to 70%, others to 40% to 50%. Begin with a once-daily application. After one to two weeks, experiment with twice daily if relief is insufficient and skin tolerance is good. Many find five days on, two days off works well.

If treating multiple chronic areas, rotate application sites daily rather than treating everything simultaneously. This prevents cumulative skin exposure while maintaining therapeutic coverage. Take a full week off every three to five weeks to assess whether the underlying condition is improving.

Region-Specific Application Guides

Lower back (lumbar region): Use 60% to 70% DMSO in aloe vera gel or coconut oil. Cover the entire lumbar spine from the bottom of the ribcage to the top of the buttocks, extending two to five inches on either side. Use a large cotton pad (4x4 inches) or paint roller applicator for even coverage. Use 5 to 6 milliliters (approximately one teaspoon). Focus on muscular areas on either side of the spine, not directly over the spine itself.

Shoulders (deltoid and rotator cuff): Use 50% to 60% DMSO in aloe vera gel. Cover the entire shoulder cap, extending to the upper neck-shoulder junction and down the upper arm two to five inches. Use clean hands or a medium cotton pad. Use 2 to 3 milliliters per shoulder. Apply 30 to 45 minutes before shoulder mobility exercises or physical therapy. Avoid the armpit area due to thin, sensitive skin.

Calves and lower legs: Use 60% to 70% DMSO in aloe vera gel or coconut oil. For calf strains, cover the entire calf from behind the knee to above the ankle. For shin splints, focus on the front of the lower leg along the shin bone. Use 3 to 5 milliliters per calf. Elevate the leg for 15 to 20 minutes after DMSO application to enhance circulation and reduce swelling.

Complementary Recovery Strategies

Ice-DMSO protocol: Apply ice pack for 15 to 20 minutes, remove ice and wait 10 to 15 minutes, apply DMSO, wait 30 minutes for absorption, then reapply ice if swelling is severe.

Compression-DMSO protocol: Apply DMSO, wait 30 to 45 minutes for complete absorption, apply compression wrap, keep compression on for 2 to 5 hours or overnight, remove compression and allow skin to breathe for several hours before next DMSO application. Never apply compression immediately after DMSO. This can drive DMSO deeper than intended or increase irritation risk.

Red-Flag Symptoms Requiring Medical Attention

Seek immediate medical attention if the injured area swells dramatically or develops extensive bruising (suggests significant muscle tearing or internal bleeding), you heard or felt a pop during injury, have visible deformity, or cannot contract the muscle at all (likely significant or complete tear), pain remains at same level or worsens after 7 to 10 days despite consistent DMSO use and conservative measures (imaging may be needed), or the area becomes increasingly red, hot, or you develop fever (signs of infection).

Taming Inflammation: DMSO for Tendonitis, Bursitis, and Swelling

Inflammatory conditions like tendonitis, bursitis, and localized swelling are notoriously stubborn. DMSO's potent anti-inflammatory properties make it particularly valuable for these conditions, but success requires precise application techniques and patience.

Inflammation-Specific Protocols

Acute flare-ups: Start with 60% DMSO in aloe vera gel. Avoid exceeding 70% even for acute conditions on sensitive areas like wrists or elbows. Apply three times daily for the first 48 to 72 hours, spacing applications six to eight hours apart.

Apply directly to the point of maximum tenderness plus a two-inch radius around it. For tendonitis, cover the tendon's entire path from muscle to bone insertion. For bursitis, cover the entire bursa area, which may be larger than the pain suggests.

Maintain three times daily for three to five days maximum, then reduce to twice daily as inflammation subsides. Combine DMSO with strict rest. DMSO reduces pain, which can tempt you to resume aggravating activities too soon. The pain relief is therapeutic, but the underlying inflammation still needs time to resolve.

Chronic inflammatory conditions: Start with 50% DMSO in aloe vera gel or coconut oil. You'll be using DMSO long-term, so starting with a moderate concentration allows room to increase if needed while minimizing cumulative skin irritation.

Apply twice daily, morning and evening, for the first two to three weeks. After this initial period, reassess. Many chronic conditions respond well to maintenance dosing of once daily or five days per week after initial improvement.

Use DMSO for three to five weeks continuously, then take a three to five-day break. During the break, assess your true baseline. Has the inflammation improved, or was DMSO merely masking symptoms? Resume DMSO and repeat this cycle until the condition resolves or plateaus.

Condition-specific guidance: For tendonitis (Achilles, rotator cuff, tennis elbow, De Quervain's), follow the tendon's entire path. For Achilles tendonitis, apply from the calf muscle insertion down to the heel bone attachment. For tennis elbow, cover the outer elbow and extend two to three inches down the forearm. DMSO's pain relief can mask tendon damage and lead to rupture if you return to aggravating activities too soon.

For bursitis (shoulder, elbow, hip, knee), cover the entire swollen area. Bursae can extend several inches. If the bursa area is hot, increasingly red, or you develop a fever, stop DMSO immediately and seek medical care. Infected bursitis requires antibiotics.

Application Around Sensitive, Mobile Areas

Wrists: Start with 30% DMSO, increasing to 50% only after one week of good tolerance. Use a cotton swab for precise application. For De Quervain's, apply along the affected tendons on the thumb side. For wrist inflammation, apply to the top of the wrist, avoiding the more sensitive palm side.

Consider applying a thin layer of petroleum jelly or coconut oil to the surrounding unaffected skin before DMSO application. This creates a protective barrier. Apply DMSO when you can rest the wrist for 30 to 45 minutes. Evening is often best.

Elbows: Use 50% to 60% DMSO in aloe vera gel. For tennis elbow (lateral epicondylitis), apply to the outer elbow bump and two to three inches down the forearm. For golfer's elbow (medial epicondylitis), apply to the inner elbow bump. The inner elbow crease has very thin skin. If treating golfer's elbow, protect the elbow crease with petroleum jelly before DMSO application. Keep elbow slightly bent during application and for 30 minutes after.

Ankles: Use 60% DMSO in aloe vera gel. For Achilles tendonitis, apply along the entire tendon from the calf to the heel using light pressure. For ankle sprains, cover the swollen area generously, usually the outer ankle. Elevate the ankle for 20 to 30 minutes after DMSO application.

Progress Monitoring Checklists

Track daily: pain at rest (0-10 scale), pain with specific aggravating movement, visible swelling (measure if applicable), range of motion limitations, and stiffness duration (especially morning stiffness).

Expect gradual improvement over a few weeks. Tendonitis and bursitis rarely resolve quickly. If you see no improvement after three weeks of appropriate DMSO use, the protocol may need adjustment or the condition may require a different intervention.

Unique Risks: Pain Masking and Overuse

DMSO's pain relief can mask underlying damage and lead to overuse injuries. Use pain reduction for therapeutic movement (gentle stretching, physical therapy), not return to sport or aggravating activities. If inflammation worsens or new symptoms develop (numbness, weakness), stop DMSO and consult a healthcare provider.

Tension Headache & Migraine Relief: Safe Use on Neck and Temples

Headaches present unique DMSO challenges because you're applying to sensitive facial and neck areas with thin skin and rich blood supply. Conservative concentrations and careful technique are non-negotiable.

Low-Dilution Protocols for Sensitive Areas

Tension headaches: Use 25% to 30% DMSO in aloe vera gel. Never exceed 40% on face, neck, or scalp, regardless of tolerance elsewhere. Apply to the posterior neck at the base of the skull, where neck muscles attach, temples using very light application, or forehead (avoiding eye area completely). Use only a few drops (2 to 5 drops total). Apply with a cotton swab for precise placement.

Apply at headache onset, not as preventive treatment. If the headache doesn't improve within two to four hours, you can apply a second time, but avoid repeated applications throughout the day. Never use DMSO multiple times daily as headache prevention.

Migraines: Use 15% to 25% DMSO in aloe vera gel. Migraine sufferers often have heightened sensitivity during attacks, requiring gentler treatment. Apply to the same areas as tension headaches, but with extra caution. Some find DMSO helpful during the prodrome phase before severe pain develops, others during the headache phase. Experiment cautiously to find your pattern.

Site Selection Decision Tree

Choose application sites based on where you feel tension or pain most intensely:

- Neck-based tension headaches? Focus on the posterior neck
- Temple-focused headaches? Apply to temples with extreme care to avoid eye contact
- Forehead pressure? Apply to the forehead, but stay well clear of eyebrows and eyes

Never apply near the eyes, mouth, nose, or on broken skin.

Supportive Measures for Holistic Management

Combine DMSO with proven headache relief strategies: Apply in a dark, quiet room to minimize sensory triggers. Use a cold compress on the forehead or neck for 15 minutes, then apply DMSO. Practice deep breathing or meditation 20 to 30 minutes after DMSO application when pain relief begins. Ensure adequate hydration. Avoid headache triggers for 24 hours after DMSO use (alcohol, caffeine withdrawal, bright lights, strong odors).

Tracking Headache Patterns

Maintain headache log noting: date and time of onset, suspected triggers, headache type and location, DMSO concentration used, amount applied and where, time from DMSO application to relief (if any), duration of relief, and any side effects.

After tracking two to four weeks, review for patterns. Does DMSO work better for tension versus migraine? Is there an optimal concentration? Does application timing matter? Use this data to refine your approach.

Post-Injury and Post-Surgery Recovery: Enhancing Healing and Comfort

DMSO can support recovery after injury or surgery, but integration with medical care requires careful coordination and conservative protocols to avoid interfering with healing.

Integration Guidelines with Medical Care

Never begin DMSO after surgery without discussing it with your surgeon. Surgical wounds require specific healing timelines, and DMSO's effects on this process aren't fully studied. Most surgeons recommend waiting until incisions are completely healed with intact skin (typically three to four weeks minimum).

When your surgeon approves DMSO, start conservatively with 40% to 50% concentration regardless of tolerance elsewhere. Apply only to areas of pain or swelling, not directly on or near healing incisions. Never apply to areas with surgical drains, staples, or sutures in place. If you develop any signs of infection (redness, warmth, swelling, drainage, fever), stop DMSO immediately and contact your surgical team.

Supportive Routines for Recovery

Post-surgical swelling and bruising: Apply DMSO once or twice daily to swollen areas, maintaining a two-inch distance from incisions. Use a conservative 40% to 50% concentration. Combine with elevation and gentle compression as directed by your surgical team. Continue for two to four weeks or until swelling resolves.

Post-surgical pain management: Apply DMSO to painful areas after the acute post-operative period (typically one to two weeks post-surgery). Use as an adjunct to prescribed pain medications, not a replacement. Discuss any changes in pain medication needs with your surgeon.

Post-Surgical Scar Considerations

Wait until incisions are completely healed and sutures or staples are removed (typically four to six weeks post-surgery). Use 50% to 60% DMSO in vitamin E oil or aloe vera gel. Apply directly to scar tissue once daily, massaging gently for one to two minutes. Continue for three to six months for optimal scar remodeling.

Monitoring Checklist for Safe Post-Surgical Use

Before each application, verify:

- No signs of infection at the surgical site
- Incisions fully healed with no scabbing or drainage
- No fever or systemic signs of infection

- Adequate time has passed since surgery, per the surgeon's guidance

After application, monitor for:

- Any increased warmth, redness, or swelling at surgical sites
- Any reopening of healed incisions
- Any unusual drainage or odor
- Any systemic symptoms (fever, malaise)

If any concerning signs develop, stop DMSO and contact your surgical team immediately.

Chapter Six

Creating Custom DMSO Blends and Solving Common Problems

Most people start DMSO use with pre-diluted products or simple mixtures following basic recipes. As you gain experience and understand your body's response, you'll likely want to customize formulations for specific needs, experiment with different carriers, or troubleshoot issues that arise. This chapter helps you move from simply following recipes to creating blends that fit your condition, skin type, and everyday routine. You'll learn which carrier agents enhance DMSO's effects, how to prepare custom dilutions safely, when and how to combine DMSO with other therapeutic substances, and how to solve problems when your current protocol isn't working optimally.

Choosing the Right Carrier Agents: Aloe, Distilled Water, and Beyond

DMSO is rarely used at full strength. The carrier agent you mix with it determines not only how gentle the application will be, but also how it feels on your skin, how quickly it absorbs, and how effective it is for your specific condition.

Why Carriers Do More Than Just Dilute

Carrier agents serve multiple critical functions. They reduce skin irritation by bringing DMSO concentration down to levels your skin can tolerate while maintaining therapeutic benefits. They improve spreadability, transforming viscous, sticky DMSO into smooth, evenly applied solutions. Some carriers provide complementary benefits. Aloe vera soothes inflamed skin. Magnesium oil relaxes muscles. Coconut oil moisturizes. The right carrier enhances DMSO's effectiveness through synergistic action.

Carriers also control the absorption rate. Water-based carriers allow rapid absorption, ideal when you need to dress quickly. Oil-based carriers slow absorption, providing extended contact time for chronic conditions requiring sustained delivery.

Popular Carriers Compared: Pros, Cons, and Best Uses

Distilled water serves as the universal dilutant. It's readily available, inexpensive, mixes completely with DMSO, and allows for the fastest absorption. Water-based DMSO dries quickly, making it practical for daytime use or large body areas. The downside: no moisturizing benefit, can be drying with repeated use, and has a shorter shelf life than oil-based blends. Best for large muscle groups (back, thighs, calves), acute injuries where rapid absorption is desired, and when you need to dress quickly after application. Typical dilution: 50% to 70% DMSO in distilled water.

Aloe vera gel provides soothing, anti-inflammatory properties that enhance DMSO's effects. It moisturizes, preventing dryness from repeated DMSO use, and spreads easily with a pleasant texture. The disadvantages: higher cost than water, requires pure aloe without alcohol or fragrances, slight stickiness until absorbed, and potential for microbial growth if contaminated. Best for arthritic joints (especially hands and knees), sunburned or irritated skin, facial applications, dry skin, and inflammatory conditions. Typical dilution: 30% to 70% DMSO in aloe vera gel. Choose pure aloe vera gel (98% to 99% aloe from the inner leaf). Many "aloe gels" contain mostly water, thickeners, and preservatives.

Natural oils (coconut, jojoba, sweet almond, olive) provide excellent moisturization for very dry skin. Slower absorption provides extended contact time. Some oils have antimicrobial properties and a long shelf life. The greasy texture requires time to absorb and can stain clothing. DMSO doesn't mix as completely with oils, requiring vigorous shaking. Oils may clog pores on acne-prone skin. Best for chronic conditions requiring sustained delivery, very dry or mature skin, evening applications, and enhancing penetration of fat-soluble compounds. Typical dilution: 40% to 60% DMSO in carrier oil. DMSO and oil separate naturally. Shake thoroughly before each use.

Magnesium oil (magnesium chloride dissolved in water) relaxes muscles and may enhance DMSO's pain-relieving effects while addressing magnesium deficiency transdermally. It has synergistic effects for muscle cramps and mixes completely with DMSO. Disadvantages: potential stinging on sensitive skin, slight residue, higher cost, and possible itching in magnesium-sensitive individuals. Best for muscle cramps and spasms, fibromyalgia, chronic muscle tension, tension headaches, and suspected magnesium deficiency. Typical approach: 50/50 blend of DMSO solution with magnesium oil (for example, 30% DMSO solution mixed with equal parts magnesium oil creates approximately 15% final DMSO concentration).

Matching Carriers to Application Sites and Skin Types

Sensitive areas (face, neck, inner arms): Choose aloe vera gel for soothing properties. If aloe causes stickiness, use distilled water, but follow with a light moisturizer 30 minutes after DMSO absorbs.

Large muscle areas (back, thighs): Distilled water provides cost-effective coverage and quick absorption. If skin becomes dry with repeated use, switch to aloe or apply moisturizer between sessions.

Dry or mature skin: Prefer natural oils (coconut, jojoba) or aloe. These provide moisturization that counteracts DMSO's drying tendency.

Oily or acne-prone skin: Stick with water-based solutions (distilled water, aloe, witch hazel). Oils may worsen breakouts.

Sun-damaged or irritated skin: Aloe vera gel is ideal for UV-damaged tissue and provides cooling comfort.

Quick-dry needs: Distilled water absorbs fastest, allowing you to dress within 20 to 30 minutes.

Carriers to Avoid for Safety

Never use petroleum jelly or mineral oil. These petroleum-derived products may contain impurities that DMSO carries through your skin. Never use scented lotions or creams. Synthetic fragrances contain phthalates and chemicals with potential hormone-disrupting effects. Avoid chemical-laden skin creams. Commercial lotions often contain parabens, sodium lauryl sulfate, synthetic colors, and additives that become concerning when DMSO carries them through the skin barrier.

Never use essential oils at high concentrations as the primary carrier. This risks severe irritation and potential toxicity. Avoid alcohol-containing products. DMSO carries ethanol through the skin, potentially causing systemic alcohol absorption and increased irritation. Never mix DMSO with prescription or over-the-counter medication creams unless explicitly directed by a healthcare provider. DMSO alters medication absorption, potentially causing overdose or unexpected effects.

The golden rule: if you wouldn't be comfortable eating a substance or applying it to broken skin, don't mix it with DMSO. DMSO's penetration enhancement means whatever you mix with it goes into your body, not just onto your skin.

Step-by-Step Dilution Recipes for Common Uses

Having precise, tested recipes eliminates guesswork and ensures consistent results. These formulations provide exact measurements for the most common DMSO applications.

Recipe Cards for Common Conditions

Arthritis Relief for Hands (40% DMSO in Aloe):

- 4 mL pharmaceutical-grade DMSO
- 6 mL pure aloe vera gel
- Total: 10 mL
- Application: 3-5 drops per affected joint, once or twice daily

Why this formula: Lower concentration protects thin hand skin. Aloe soothes joint inflammation and prevents dryness.

Arthritis Relief for Knees (70% DMSO in Aloe):

- 14 mL pharmaceutical-grade DMSO
- 6 mL pure aloe vera gel
- Total: 20 mL
- Application: 2-3 mL per knee, once or twice daily

Why this formula: Higher concentration penetrates thick knee skin and deeper tissue to reach the joint capsule. Aloe prevents dryness.

Muscle Pain for Back and Shoulders (60% DMSO in Water):

- 18 mL pharmaceutical-grade DMSO
- 12 mL distilled water
- Total: 30 mL
- Application: 4-6 mL to the affected area, once or twice daily

Why this formula: Water-based solution absorbs quickly for large areas where you need to dress soon.

Acute Injury Treatment (70% DMSO in Water):

- 21 mL pharmaceutical-grade DMSO
- 9 mL distilled water
- Total: 30 mL
- Application: 3-4 mL to the injured area, three times daily for the first 48-72 hours, then reduce frequency

Why this formula: Higher concentration and aggressive initial frequency address acute inflammation. Time-limited to prevent cumulative skin irritation.

Tension Headache Relief (25% DMSO in Aloe):

- 2.5 mL pharmaceutical-grade DMSO
- 7.5 mL pure aloe vera gel
- Total: 10 mL
- Application: 2-5 drops to temples, posterior neck, or forehead, once per headache episode

Why this formula: Very low concentration for sensitive facial and neck areas. Never exceed 30% on face or neck.

Preparation Process Essentials

Use glass containers (preferred) or HDPE plastic #2. Never use PVC plastic, metal, or containers previously used for other purposes. Add carrier to the container first, then add DMSO slowly while stirring. This order is important for water-based solutions since mixing generates heat (a normal exothermic reaction).

Mix gently but thoroughly, stirring for at least 60 seconds. Oil-based blends require vigorous shaking for 90 seconds or more since oil and DMSO resist mixing.

Maintain strict hygiene. Wash your hands thoroughly before handling DMSO. Sterilize containers by boiling glass for 10 minutes or rinsing with 70% isopropyl alcohol and air drying completely. Work on a clean surface.

Storage and Labeling Best Practices

Label every batch before storing. Include: DMSO concentration and carrier type, additional ingredients (if stacking), date prepared, intended use or body location, expiration date based on carrier type, and warnings ("external use only," "keep away from eyes").

Storage duration by carrier type: water-based blends last 2-3 weeks at room temperature (4-6 weeks refrigerated), aloe-based blends last 3-4 weeks, oil-based blends without essential oils last 2-3 months, and any blend with essential oils lasts 4-6 weeks maximum.

Store in amber glass bottles at 60-75°F, away from direct sunlight and heat. Keep tightly capped since DMSO is hygroscopic and absorbs moisture from the air, diluting your concentration.

Troubleshooting Common Blending Mistakes

Oil-based blends separate into layers. This is normal. Shake vigorously for 60 seconds before each use. Water-based solutions develop cloudiness after initial mixing. This indicates contamination. Discard and prepare a fresh solution with sterilized equipment. Sediment settles at the bottom. This suggests degradation or contamination. Discard and prepare a fresh batch. Blends develop odor beyond

DMSO's mild garlic smell (rancid, sour, musty odors). This indicates microbial contamination. Discard immediately.

Safe "Stacking": Combining DMSO with Magnesium Oil or Essential Oils

"Stacking" refers to combining DMSO with other therapeutic substances to enhance overall effectiveness. Because DMSO carries compounds through the skin barrier, it can deliver beneficial substances deeper than they would penetrate alone. This creates therapeutic possibilities but also serious risks if done improperly.

Understanding the Stacking Concept and Its Appeal

DMSO's penetration-enhancing property transforms it into a delivery vehicle for other compounds, opening doors to synergistic combinations. Magnesium oil relaxes muscles while DMSO reduces inflammation. Together, they address multiple pain mechanisms simultaneously. Peppermint essential oil provides cooling analgesic effects while DMSO carries it deeper for enhanced relief. MSM provides sulfur for connective tissue health, while DMSO enhances absorption.

Enhanced therapeutic outcomes often exceed what either substance achieves alone. Users report faster pain relief, longer-lasting effects, and improved response in resistant conditions. Reduced DMSO concentration becomes possible when stacking. You can sometimes use 30% to 40% instead of 60% to 70% and achieve equivalent results, meaning less skin irritation.

The appeal is clear, but the risks are real. DMSO doesn't discriminate. It carries beneficial compounds through your skin, but it also carries contaminants, allergens, or toxic substances. Stacking requires knowledge, caution, and strict safety protocols.

Safety Guidelines: What's Safe and What's Dangerous

Safe to stack:

Magnesium chloride oil: Excellent safety profile with a pharmaceutical-grade product. Provides transdermal magnesium, relaxes muscles. Typical ratio: 50/50 with DMSO solution (equal parts 30% DMSO solution and magnesium oil). May sting on sensitive skin. Start with a small test area.

MSM: Closely related to DMSO chemically, with a similar safety profile. Provides organic sulfur for connective tissue health. Typical ratio: 1-2 grams MSM powder dissolved in 30 mL DMSO solution (3% to 7% MSM concentration). Use pharmaceutical-grade MSM only.

Pure essential oils (properly diluted): Safe options include lavender (calming, mild analgesic), peppermint (cooling, analgesic), eucalyptus (respiratory support), frankincense (anti-inflammatory), and helichrysum (bruising, closed wounds only). Critical rule: Never exceed 2% essential oil concentration in the final DMSO blend. That's 2 drops per teaspoon of DMSO blend maximum. Always dilute essential oil in carrier oil first, then mix with DMSO solution. Never add pure essential oil directly to DMSO.

Arnica montana extract: Good safety profile for external use. Reduces bruising and provides anti-inflammatory effects. Apply arnica gel first, allow 30 minutes to dry, then apply DMSO over it. Some people are allergic to arnica. Patch test first.

Never stack with:

Never use prescription medications (topical or oral). DMSO alters absorption dramatically, potentially causing overdose. Never use synthetic fragrances or scented products. Phthalates and synthetic chemicals have unknown systemic effects when absorbed. Never use herbal tinctures or extracts with alcohol. DMSO carries ethanol through the skin. Never use untested herbal extracts. Unknown compounds have unpredictable effects when absorbed systemically. Never use capsaicin or cayenne preparations. Extreme burning and irritation result when DMSO enhances capsaicin penetration.

Popular Stack Recipes That Work

For Muscle Cramps:

- 15 mL of 30% DMSO solution
- 15 mL pharmaceutical-grade magnesium chloride oil
- Shake well before each use
- Apply 2-3 mL to the cramping muscle, and massage for 1-2 minutes
- Use 2-3 times daily

- Particularly effective before bed for nighttime cramps
- Final concentration: ~15% DMSO with therapeutic magnesium

For Tension Headaches:

- Pre-dilute: 3 drops pure peppermint essential oil in 15 mL fractionated coconut oil
- Mix with 10 mL of 30% DMSO solution in aloe vera gel
- Stir vigorously for 2 minutes
- Store in amber glass, shake before use
- Apply 3-5 drops to temples, posterior neck, or forehead using a cotton swab
- Avoid the eye area completely
- Use once per headache episode
- Final concentration: ~12% DMSO with <1% peppermint

For Joint Support:

Dissolve 1.5 grams of pharmaceutical-grade MSM powder in 30 mL of 50% DMSO solution

Stir vigorously 2-3 minutes until MSM completely dissolves

Store in an amber glass bottle

Apply 2-3 mL to affected joints once or twice daily

Massage gently 1-2 minutes

Final concentration: 50% DMSO with 5% MSM

Minimizing Risks When Stacking

Patch-test each new combination separately before applying to large areas. Apply a dime-sized amount to the inner forearm, wait 24 hours, and observe for redness, itching, rash, or burning. If there is no reaction, test on a small area of the actual treatment site, wait another 24 hours, then proceed with full application if there is still no reaction.

Never exceed 2% essential oil concentration. More concentrated doesn't mean more effective. It means a higher risk of severe irritation, chemical burns, systemic toxicity, and permanent sensitization.

Never stack more than two additional agents at once. Limit to DMSO plus carrier plus one additional active (for example, DMSO plus aloe plus magnesium). Adding multiple essential oils or combining magnesium plus MSM plus essential oils creates complexity that makes troubleshooting impossible and increases interaction risks.

Start with lower DMSO concentrations when stacking. Begin with 30% to 40% DMSO rather than 60% to 70%. Additional substances may enhance overall effectiveness, allowing lower DMSO concentration and minimized skin irritation risk.

Monitor for cumulative effects. Stacked formulations can increase both benefits and side effects. Track use carefully, noting skin changes, unusual sensations, or systemic effects like headache, nausea, or fatigue. If these develop, simplify the formula by removing additional actives and using DMSO alone.

Batch-Mixing and Storage: Keeping DIY Blends Potent and Safe

Preparing DMSO blends in larger quantities saves time and ensures consistency, but batch-mixing introduces preservation challenges that single-use mixing avoids.

Benefits and Risks of Preparing in Advance

Batch-mixing offers convenience for frequent users. If you apply DMSO daily for chronic conditions, mixing a week's or a month's supply at once eliminates daily preparation. Consistency in concentration ensures every application uses the exact same percentage. Careful measurement prevents small variations that make tracking effectiveness difficult. Time efficiency: mixing 100 mL once takes marginally longer than mixing 10 mL, but provides 10 days of treatment.

The risks include contamination vulnerability. Every time you open a container, you introduce potential contaminants (bacteria, fungi, environmental particles). Water-based blends are particularly susceptible to microbial growth. Potency degradation affects carriers like aloe vera and essential oils over time. Inflexibility: batch preparation locks you into one concentration and carrier. If you need to adjust, you must discard the batch.

Batch-mix if you use DMSO at the same concentration, same carrier, at least 5 times per week for an established condition. Continue single-use mixing if you're still experimenting with formulations, use DMSO sporadically, or treat multiple conditions requiring different concentrations.

Safe Batch Preparation: Hygiene and Protocols

Sterilize containers before use. For glass: wash with hot soapy water, boil for 10 minutes fully submerged, remove with clean tongs, air dry completely upside down on a clean towel. For HDPE plastic: wash with hot soapy water, rinse with 70% isopropyl alcohol (cannot boil), air dry completely.

Calculate quantities based on application frequency and storage life. If using 3 mL daily, prepare 50-60 mL for a 2-week supply (maximum recommended storage time for water-based blends).

Add the carrier to the sterilized container first. This allows accurate measurement before DMSO's volume is added. Add DMSO slowly while stirring continuously. For water-based solutions, expect heat generation (normal exothermic reaction). Mix thoroughly for a minimum of 60 seconds. Oil-based blends require vigorous shaking for 2-3 minutes. Allow the solution to cool to room temperature before capping. Add additional actives last (if stacking with magnesium oil, MSM, or essential oils, add after DMSO and carrier are thoroughly mixed).

Label completely before storing: exact DMSO concentration and carrier type, additional active ingredients with approximate concentrations, intended use or body location, preparation date, expiration date based on carrier type, storage instructions, and safety warnings ("external use only," "keep away from eyes").

Best Storage Practices to Maintain Potency

Use amber glass (ideal for light protection and non-reactive), clear glass (acceptable but requires dark storage location), or HDPE plastic #2 (acceptable, unbreakable, but less ideal for long-term storage).

Store at 60-75°F, avoiding temperature fluctuations. Refrigeration is optional for water-based blends and can extend life to 4-6 weeks, but it brings condensation risks. Keep in a dark location (cabinet, drawer, or opaque bag) since UV light degrades DMSO and carriers. Keep tightly capped. DMSO is hygroscopic and absorbs moisture from the air, diluting the concentration over time. Store away from children and pets with clear labeling.

Recognizing When a Blend Has Spoiled

Visual signs: color change (darkening, yellowing, brown or gray tones), cloudiness in previously clear solutions, separation that won't remix after vigorous shaking for 60 seconds, or visible particles, sediment, or floating material.

Olfactory signs: DMSO's normal mild garlic or sulfur smell is expected. Abnormal odors include rancid or sour smell (bacterial contamination), strong chemical odor unlike DMSO's typical scent (degradation), musty or moldy smell (fungal contamination), or complete loss of essential oil scent (oil has evaporated or degraded).

Discard batches after maximum storage times even without obvious spoilage: water-based after 2-3 weeks (4-6 weeks refrigerated), aloe-based after 3-4 weeks, oil-based without essential oils after 2-3 months, oil-based with essential oils after 4-6 weeks, and any blend with magnesium oil after 3-4 weeks.

When in doubt, throw it out. The cost of ingredients is trivial compared to the risk of skin infection from a contaminated product.

Troubleshooting Protocols: Adjusting for Sensitivity, Side Effects, and Non-Response

DMSO use rarely proceeds perfectly from start to finish. Skin sensitivity develops, formulas that worked suddenly cause irritation, or expected benefits fail to materialize. Knowing how to recognize problems early and adjust systematically prevents minor issues from becoming major setbacks.

Recognizing When Your Protocol Needs Adjustment

Early warning symptoms (within hours to days): Excessive redness where bright red coloration persists 3+ hours signals excessive concentration. Stinging or burning where sharp stinging intensifies rather than fades indicates the formula is too strong. Prolonged irritation where skin remains sensitive to touch hours after application means you've exceeded the tolerance threshold.

Delayed reactions (after days to weeks): Progressive dryness, where application areas become increasingly dry, flaky, or rough, predicts future irritation. Peeling or scaling indicates damage to the protective outer layer requiring immediate adjustment. Headaches, fatigue, or nausea likely indicate sensitivity or excessive dosing rather than actual detoxification and warrant reducing concentration or frequency.

Lack of improvement: If you've applied DMSO consistently at appropriate concentrations for two weeks without any improvement in pain, stiffness, or other symptoms, the current protocol isn't working. Plateaued benefits, where initial improvement is followed by stagnation, suggest you've reached maximum benefit at that concentration or frequency.

Stepwise Adjustment Strategies

If experiencing irritation, reduce concentration by 10% to 15%. From 70% reduce to 60% or 55%. From 60% reduce to 50% or 45%. From 50% reduce to 40% or 35%. Apply reduced concentration for 5-7 days. If irritation resolves, you've found a better baseline. If irritation persists, reduce another 10% and reassess.

Often, frequency is the problem, not concentration. Try reducing application frequency before lowering DMSO percentage. From 3 times daily, reduce to 2 times daily. From 2 times daily, reduce to once daily. From daily to every other day or 5 days per week. This maintains therapeutic concentration while giving skin more recovery time.

When to Suspend Use and Reintroduce DMSO

Stop all DMSO use immediately if you have persistent redness or irritation despite reducing concentration, peeling, cracking, or broken skin in the application area, development of rash or hives, or any systemic symptoms like headache, nausea, or unusual fatigue.

Allow minimum 5-7 days of complete rest (longer for severe reactions, up to 2 weeks). During break, moisturize application areas 2-3 times daily with pure aloe or unscented lotion. Monitor healing. Skin should return to its normal appearance and feel.

After full recovery, restart at 50% lower concentration than what caused the reaction. If you reacted to 60%, restart at 30%. Begin with a once every other day application. Observe for 1 week. If no reaction, increase to daily. After another week of good tolerance, consider increasing the concentration by 10% if needed for effectiveness.

Patch-test the new formula before full application. Apply a dime-sized amount to the inner forearm, wait 24 hours. Apply a small amount to the actual treatment area, wait another 24 hours. If no reaction, proceed with the full protocol.

Addressing Non-Response: When DMSO Doesn't Seem to Work

Before concluding DMSO doesn't work, verify optimal use. Are you applying to clean, dry skin? Using enough product (joints need 2-3 mL, large muscles need 4-6 mL)? Massaging it in for 30-60 seconds rather than just daubing? Using pharmaceutical-grade DMSO? Allowing adequate absorption time (20-30 minutes of air exposure)?

Some conditions don't respond to DMSO because they require different treatment. Severe arthritis with significant joint damage may need medical intervention. Nerve pain often requires different approaches than inflammatory pain. Infections require antibiotics, not DMSO. If appropriate DMSO use for 4 weeks produces zero improvement, a medical evaluation is warranted.

DMSO works best as part of a comprehensive treatment. Combine with appropriate physical therapy or exercise, address contributing factors (poor ergonomics, nutritional deficiencies), consider complementary modalities (heat/cold therapy), and explore oral supplements that work synergistically. Sometimes DMSO provides 40% improvement, and adding these approaches brings total improvement to 70-80%, better than either alone.

Protocol Customization: Adjusting Recipes for Sensitive Skin or High-Risk Areas

Standard DMSO protocols work well for most users on typical body areas, but sensitive skin, high-risk locations, and individual variations require customized approaches.

Modifying Standard Recipes for Sensitive Areas

For face, neck, inner arms, or users with reactive skin, start with ultra-gentle concentrations: 15% to 20% DMSO in soothing carrier (1.5-2 mL DMSO with 8-8.5 mL aloe vera gel for 10 mL total).

Standard sensitive-area concentration uses 25% to 30% DMSO (2.5-3 mL DMSO with 7-7.5 mL carrier for 10 mL total).

For large sensitive areas, increase carrier volume. High-carrier formula: 20% DMSO in a generous aloe base (4 mL DMSO with 16 mL aloe vera gel for 20 mL total). This provides enough volume to cover large sensitive areas like the entire face, or full neck and shoulders.

Add soothing ingredients to buffer DMSO. Aloe-calendula blend: 7 mL pure aloe vera gel, 1 mL alcohol-free calendula extract, 2 mL DMSO (creates 20% DMSO with additional anti-inflammatory properties).

Troubleshooting Common Customization Issues

If your customized formula still causes stinging or redness, dilute the existing blend by 25%. Take 7.5 mL of the current formula, add 2.5 mL pure carrier, creating 10 mL at 75% of the original concentration. Continue stepwise dilution until you find a comfortable concentration.

If irritation persists despite dilution, switch carriers. Some people tolerate aloe poorly but do well with distilled water or coconut oil. Others find water too drying, but respond well to aloe. Test the new carrier at the same or lower DMSO concentration. If switching from aloe to water, prepare a new batch at 5% to 10% lower DMSO concentration to account for water's faster absorption. If switching from water to oil, prepare at the same concentration but expect slower absorption, requiring longer wait times before dressing.

If uncertain which variable causes problems (concentration, carrier, or frequency), simplify to baseline. Use 20% DMSO in distilled water once every other day. If this causes no irritation, you've found your starting point. Gradually add back variables one at a time.

Special Considerations for Age, Skin Type, and Allergic History

For older adults or those with thin skin, test on a small area first, start at the lowest concentrations (15% to 20%), increase very gradually (5% increments instead of 10%), and take frequent breaks (one day off per week minimum).

For those with a history of allergic reactions to topical products, perform an extended patch test (48 to 72 hours instead of 24), start with a single-ingredient carrier (distilled water only, no aloe or oils initially), avoid all essential oils and botanical extracts until you've established DMSO tolerance, and keep detailed notes of any reactions for pattern identification.

Avoid essential oils on broken or compromised skin. These can cause severe irritation when the skin barrier is damaged.

Decision-Making Flowchart for Protocol Adjustments

Follow this systematic approach when experiencing problems:

Step 1: Is the problem irritation (redness, stinging, burning)?

YES → Reduce concentration by 10% to 15%. Wait 5 to 7 days. Problem resolved? If YES, continue at a lower concentration. If NO, go to Step 2.

NO → Go to Step 5.

Step 2: Does irritation persist at reduced concentration?

YES → Reduce frequency (from 2x daily to 1x daily, or from daily to every other day). Wait 5 to 7 days. Problem resolved? If YES, continue at a lower frequency. If NO, go to Step 3.

NO → Continue at reduced concentration.

Step 3: Does irritation persist despite lower concentration and frequency?

YES → Switch carrier. Try a different carrier at the same or lower concentration. Wait 5 to 7 days. Problem resolved? If YES, continue with the new carrier. If NO, go to Step 4.

NO → Continue current protocol.

Step 4: Does irritation persist despite all adjustments?

YES → Stop DMSO use for 5 to 7 days. Allow complete skin recovery. After recovery, restart at 50% lower concentration than the original with a different carrier. Still problematic? DMSO may not be appropriate for you. Consult a healthcare provider.

Step 5: Is the problem a lack of effectiveness (no symptom improvement)?

YES → Verify you're using pharmaceutical-grade DMSO, applying to clean, dry skin, using an adequate amount, massaging for 30 to 60 seconds, and allowing 20 to 30 minutes absorption time. All verified? If YES and still no improvement after 4 weeks, consult a healthcare provider for alternative treatments. If NO, correct application technique and reassess after 2 weeks.

Golden rules for all adjustments: Change only one variable at a time (concentration OR frequency OR carrier, never multiple simultaneously). Wait 5 to 7 days between changes to observe true effects. Keep detailed notes of what you tried and the results observed. If uncertain at any point, err on the side of caution and use lower concentrations.

Chapter Seven

Advanced DMSO: What Works for Pets, What's Experimental, and What to Avoid

DMSO's versatility extends beyond the foundational protocols you've learned. While the previous chapters equipped you with essential skills for safe, effective use, certain situations require specialized knowledge. This chapter addresses advanced applications, including off-label uses where evidence exists but FDA approval doesn't, adapting DMSO protocols for animals, combining DMSO with other treatments safely, and learning from others' mistakes to avoid common pitfalls. These topics demand extra caution and often benefit from professional oversight, but they represent important extensions of DMSO's therapeutic potential when approached responsibly.

Beyond FDA Approval: What Actually Works and What's Just Hope

DMSO's versatility extends far beyond its single FDA-approved use, yet navigating off-label applications requires understanding where solid evidence exists and where you're venturing into uncertain territory.

What "Off-Label" and "Experimental" Actually Mean

"Off-label" use refers to employing a medication or substance for purposes not explicitly approved by regulatory authorities like the FDA. For DMSO, the only FDA-approved indication is interstitial cystitis treated via bladder instillation. Every other use, whether arthritis, muscle pain, or headaches, is technically off-label even when substantial evidence and decades of clinical experience support it.

"Experimental" uses go further, representing applications with minimal scientific study, often based on DMSO's known properties and theoretical benefits. The distinction matters because off-label uses with robust evidence carry relatively low risk when approached properly, while experimental uses with minimal data carry unknown risks and unpredictable outcomes.

Legal context matters too. In the United States and most countries, off-label use of approved substances is legal. Patient self-use of pharmaceutical-grade DMSO for off-label purposes occupies a legal gray area, not explicitly illegal but without regulatory oversight or protection.

Where Evidence Actually Exists

Interstitial cystitis stands alone with FDA approval. Treatment involves bladder instillations performed by a urologist, using 50% DMSO solution instilled directly into the bladder via catheter in a series of four to eight weekly treatments. Research shows 50% to 70% of patients experience meaningful symptom relief.

Scleroderma, an autoimmune disease causing skin and organ hardening, has moderate evidence for topical DMSO use. Research from the 1960s through 1980s explored DMSO at 70% to 90% concentrations for skin manifestations. Several small trials showed DMSO softened hardened skin and improved flexibility in some patients, though results were inconsistent. For a condition as serious as scleroderma, DMSO should only be considered under medical supervision as part of comprehensive disease management.

Nerve pain represents another area where DMSO has been explored with limited but intriguing results. Complex regional pain syndrome has been the focus of most research attention, with a few small studies suggesting topical DMSO may help some patients. For other neuropathic pain types like diabetic neuropathy or post-herpetic neuralgia, evidence is largely anecdotal. Neuropathic pain is notoriously difficult to treat, and DMSO works best as one component of multimodal pain management rather than a standalone solution.

Wound healing and burn treatment have been investigated primarily in veterinary medicine and research settings outside the United States. Some animal studies and small human trials suggest DMSO can reduce healing time, though large-scale human trials are lacking. Critical safety note: never apply DMSO to open wounds or fresh burns without explicit medical supervision. DMSO carries bacteria from the skin surface deep into wounds, dramatically increasing infection risk.

Understanding Risks and Uncertainties

The lack of extensive research on many DMSO applications doesn't necessarily mean they don't work. It often means pharmaceutical companies have no financial incentive to fund expensive clinical trials for an unpatentable substance. Absence of evidence isn't evidence of absence, but it does mean you're venturing into territory where outcomes are unpredictable and risks incompletely characterized.

Long-term safety data for many applications simply doesn't exist. Most DMSO research involves short-term use (weeks to months), not years of continuous application. Potential cumulative effects, interactions with aging, or impacts on specific organ systems remain unclear.

For serious medical conditions like autoimmune diseases, neurological disorders, or cancer, DMSO should never replace proven medical treatment. If you want to add DMSO to your regimen, inform your physician. Continue standard medical care, establish clear monitoring parameters with your healthcare team, and be prepared to stop if your condition worsens.

Responsible Experimentation Guidelines

If you choose to explore experimental DMSO applications, start conservatively. Use low concentrations (30% to 40%), apply to small areas initially, increase slowly only if you tolerate treatment well and see some benefit, and document everything. Track not just the symptom you're targeting but overall health indicators, sleep quality, energy levels, and any unexpected changes.

Consider working with integrative medicine practitioners familiar with DMSO. These providers can offer guidance, monitor your progress, and help distinguish between beneficial effects, placebo responses, and concerning reactions.

Helping Your Pet: DMSO for Joint Pain in Dogs and Horses

DMSO has been part of veterinary medicine longer than human medicine, with a stronger regulatory foundation and broader acceptance. For horse owners and dog guardians seeking alternatives to long-term NSAIDs for chronic pain, veterinary-grade DMSO offers a well-established option.

DMSO's Role in Veterinary Medicine

Unlike human medicine, where DMSO has only one FDA-approved use, veterinary DMSO enjoys broader acceptance. The FDA approved DMSO specifically for horses in the 1970s for reducing acute swelling due to trauma.

In equine medicine, DMSO addresses acute joint inflammation, particularly in fetlock, hock, and knee joints. Laminitis, the devastating hoof inflammation that can end a horse's career, often involves DMSO as part of comprehensive treatment. Soft tissue injuries, including tendon and ligament strains, respond well to DMSO's anti-inflammatory effects.

For dogs, DMSO use is technically off-label but increasingly common. Veterinarians familiar with equine medicine have adapted protocols for canine patients, particularly large-breed dogs suffering from hip or elbow dysplasia. DMSO offers an alternative to long-term NSAID use with its kidney damage and gastrointestinal bleeding risks.

Species-Specific Protocols and Dosing

Horses tolerate higher concentrations due to large muscle mass and thick skin. The commercial 90% DMSO gel formulated for equine use represents standard treatment. Apply 20 to 40 milliliters for legs or 30 to 60 milliliters for large muscle areas, massaging gently for two to three minutes. For horses with sensitive skin or prolonged treatment, dilute to 70%.

Frequency depends on acute versus chronic conditions. Fresh injuries benefit from applications two to three times daily for three to five days, then reduce to twice daily. Chronic conditions often do well with once or twice daily application with periodic breaks (five days on, two days off).

Dogs require different approaches due to their smaller size, thinner skin, and strong licking instinct. Use 50% to 70% concentration rather than the 90% gel used in horses. Volumes are much smaller, scaled to dog size: toy breeds under 25 pounds receive only two milliliters, while large breeds over 60 pounds might get five milliliters for hip applications.

Application location matters because skin thickness varies dramatically. Thick skin over the hips and shoulders tolerates DMSO better than thin-skinned belly, inner legs, or face. The licking problem requires creative solutions: distraction with play or treats, direct supervision during the 20 to 30 minutes needed for absorption, or temporary use of an Elizabethan collar if the dog cannot be redirected.

Safety Guidelines and Veterinary Consultation

Never use industrial-grade DMSO on animals. Only use pharmaceutical or veterinary-grade DMSO clearly labeled for animal use. Diagnosis must precede treatment. What appears to be simple arthritis could be bone cancer, Lyme disease, immune-mediated joint disease, or a fracture. Veterinary evaluation establishes what you're treating.

Watch for adverse reactions. Skin irritation is most common, ranging from mild redness to significant dermatitis requiring discontinuation. Unlike humans, animals show discomfort through behavior: increased resistance to application, attempting to bite or scratch at treated areas, or general behavioral changes.

Owner Responsibilities and Monitoring

Animals cannot consent to treatment or clearly communicate subtle side effects, placing extra responsibility on you to monitor carefully. Daily monitoring should include examining application sites for skin changes, assessing your animal's comfort during application, and tracking whether the condition actually improves.

Store veterinary DMSO in clearly labeled containers in secure locations where animals cannot access it. Keep away from food preparation areas and animal food and water storage. For animals involved in performance or competition, check governing body rules regarding DMSO use and discontinue at appropriate times before competition (usually 48 to 72 hours minimum).

DMSO and Other Treatments: What's Safe to Combine and What's Dangerous

DMSO's ability to enhance skin penetration creates both opportunities and risks when combined with other substances. Understanding which combinations carry acceptable risks and which venture into dangerous territory is essential for safe use.

Why People Combine Treatments

DMSO temporarily disrupts the skin's protective barrier, creating channels through which other substances pass far more easily than normal. Curcumin, with notoriously poor absorption, might achieve therapeutic tissue levels when mixed with DMSO. Magnesium relaxes muscles while DMSO reduces inflammation, potentially addressing pain through multiple mechanisms.

These synergistic possibilities are real, but so are the risks. DMSO carries whatever is on your skin deeper into the tissue without discrimination. Therapeutic compounds get enhanced delivery, but so do contaminants, allergens, and substances that should never penetrate beyond the skin surface. More concerning, DMSO can alter the absorption and effects of prescription medications unpredictably.

Safe Supplement Combinations

MSM sits at the top of the safe combination list. Chemically, MSM is essentially DMSO with an added oxygen molecule. Dissolve one to two grams of MSM powder in 30 milliliters of 50% DMSO solution, creating a three to seven percent MSM concentration that addresses inflammation while supporting cartilage health.

Magnesium oil combines well with DMSO for muscle-related pain. Mix equal parts 30% DMSO solution and magnesium chloride oil for muscle cramps, spasms, or chronic tension. The safety profile is generally good, though magnesium oil can sting on sensitive skin.

Arnica can be combined through a specific technique: apply arnica gel first, wait 30 minutes for partial absorption, then apply 50% to 60% DMSO over the arnica-treated area. Use this sequence twice daily for acute injuries. Never use arnica on open wounds.

Critical Drug Interaction Warnings

Blood thinners demand absolute caution. Medications like warfarin, apixaban, rivaroxaban, aspirin, and clopidogrel reduce blood clotting. DMSO has mild anticoagulant properties. While topical DMSO alone is unlikely to cause bleeding problems, combining it with prescription anticoagulants theoretically increases bleeding risk. If you take blood thinners and want to use DMSO, inform your prescribing physician and monitor for unusual bruising, bleeding gums, or blood in urine or stool.

Insulin and diabetes medications create risk through enhanced absorption. If DMSO drove insulin deeper than intended, severe hypoglycemia could result. Wash your hands thoroughly after DMSO application before handling diabetes medications. Never apply DMSO to or near insulin injection sites. Monitor blood sugar more frequently if using DMSO regularly.

Corticosteroid creams present dangerous combinations. Topical steroids are designed for surface anti-inflammatory effects with minimal systemic absorption. DMSO destroys this design by driving steroids deeper into tissue and bloodstream, potentially causing systemic effects including immune suppression, elevated blood sugar, and bone thinning. Never apply DMSO over steroid creams or apply steroid creams over areas where you've used DMSO within 12 hours.

Practical Combination Guidelines

Never start DMSO and a new medication simultaneously. If starting new prescription medication, let it stabilize for two to four weeks before introducing DMSO. If starting DMSO, use it for two to three weeks before adding new supplements.

When combining, start more conservatively than you would with DMSO alone. Use lower concentrations (40% to 50%) and begin with every-other-day application. Maintain a comprehensive medication and supplement log, including everything you take, DMSO concentration and frequency, and dates of any changes. Review weekly and bring to all medical appointments.

Boost Your Therapy Results: Using DMSO with PT, Massage, and Acupuncture

DMSO works best not as a standalone treatment but as part of comprehensive therapeutic approaches. When thoughtfully integrated with physical therapy, massage, or acupuncture, DMSO can enhance effectiveness while these modalities address underlying issues DMSO alone cannot fix.

Benefits of Integration

Physical therapy often fails not because exercises are wrong but because pain prevents proper execution. You compensate for painful movement, developing poor patterns that perpetuate problems.

DMSO applied 30 to 45 minutes before physical therapy creates a window of reduced pain during which you can execute therapeutic movements with better form.

Massage therapy benefits similarly. Chronically tight muscles often resist skilled massage because underlying inflammation keeps them in protective spasm. DMSO applied 20 to 30 minutes before massage allows therapists to work deeper and more effectively.

Timing and Sequencing

For physical therapy sessions, apply DMSO 30 to 45 minutes before appointments. Use moderate concentration, typically 50% to 60%, for most body areas. After physical therapy, wait at least two hours before applying DMSO again. The exercises create beneficial inflammation as part of healing, and immediately suppressing this response could interfere with adaptive changes.

For massage therapy, timing depends on the massage type. For deep tissue or therapeutic massage focused on chronic tension, apply DMSO 20 to 30 minutes before sessions. For relaxation or Swedish massage, DMSO application afterward often works better, addressing areas the therapist identified as particularly problematic.

Safety Cautions and Best Practices

Your physical therapist, massage therapist, or acupuncturist needs to know you're using DMSO. Be specific about concentration, frequency, and application areas. Therapists using topical products need to know that DMSO will enhance the absorption of anything applied to the skin.

Physical therapists sometimes use heat therapy. Heat increases blood flow and enhances absorption. DMSO already enhances absorption. The combination can drive DMSO systemically at higher levels than intended. If your physical therapist plans to use heat, either skip DMSO application before that session or ensure at least four hours have passed since application.

Cautionary Tales: Real Mistakes and How to Avoid Them

Understanding what can go wrong and why helps you avoid repeating others' errors. These scenarios, based on user reports, illustrate preventable mistakes.

Real-Life DMSO Mistakes

A runner with chronic knee pain applied 99% DMSO undiluted to both knees twice daily. Within three days, the skin became bright red, hot, and began peeling. Damage took three weeks to heal. The lesson: Start with 50% to 60% dilution for knees, apply once daily initially, and reduce concentration immediately if significant stinging or redness occurs.

Someone took industrial DMSO home from a manufacturing facility for arthritic hands. After a single application, hands developed severe burning, blistering, and a chemical odor. Treatment required antibiotics, with healing taking six weeks. The lesson: Never use industrial-grade DMSO. Only pharmaceutical or veterinary-grade DMSO belongs on your body.

An individual mixed DMSO with multiple essential oils for headaches, totaling an eight percent essential oil concentration. Within an hour, nausea, dizziness, and a severe headache developed. The lesson: Never exceed two percent total essential oil concentration, and always patch test custom blends.

Someone applied DMSO to a slow-healing leg cut, hoping to speed recovery. The wound became infected within 48 hours, requiring antibiotics. The lesson: Wait until wounds completely close with intact skin before using DMSO anywhere near them.

Prevention and Mistake-Proofing

Prevention requires consistently following basic principles: Always verify the pharmaceutical grade before purchase. Start with appropriate concentrations for body area (30% to 50% for sensitive areas, 50% to 70% for standard areas). Patch test all new formulations for 24 to 48 hours. Never apply to broken skin, open wounds, or mucous membranes. Adjust immediately when warning signs appear (persistent redness, stinging, burning).

If you do make a mistake, stop DMSO use immediately. Wash the affected area thoroughly with mild soap and cool water. Apply cool compresses for skin irritation. Monitor for signs of infection (increasing redness, warmth, pus, fever). Seek medical attention if symptoms are severe or don't improve within 24 to 48 hours.

Before reintroducing DMSO after a negative experience, allow complete skin healing (minimum 5 to 7 days). Restart at 50% lower concentration than what caused the reaction. Begin with a once every other day application. Observe for one week before increasing frequency. If problems recur, DMSO may not be appropriate for you.

Chapter Eight

Getting Your Doctor on Board: How to Talk About DMSO Without Getting Dismissed

Walking into your doctor's office and announcing you're using DMSO can go one of two ways. Either you'll encounter a provider who's intrigued and willing to discuss it, or you'll face skepticism ranging from mild concern to outright dismissal. The outcome often depends less on your doctor's personality than on how you present the information. Preparation transforms what could be a defensive confrontation into productive collaboration.

What to Bring to Your Appointment: Data, Evidence, and Smart Questions

Most physicians have heard of DMSO in passing, perhaps during medical school in a lecture on unusual therapies. Few have prescribed it, fewer still have studied current research, and many harbor outdated concerns from decades-old safety debates.

Walking in unprepared, mentioning DMSO casually, and hoping your doctor will fill in the knowledge gaps rarely works. The appointment time is limited, your doctor has other patients waiting, and expecting them to research DMSO on the spot isn't realistic.

Why Preparation Changes Everything

Coming prepared demonstrates you've done serious homework rather than latching onto an internet cure. It shows respect for your provider's time by bringing the information they'd need to evaluate DMSO. Most importantly, it shifts the conversation from "Should I try this random thing I read about?" to "I've researched this approach and would like your input on whether it fits my situation."

Bring your symptom logs showing what you've tracked, how long you've experienced the problem, and what other treatments you've tried. Include treatment records documenting DMSO use if you've already started, including concentrations, frequency, application sites, and any side effects or benefits observed. Compile a complete list of current medications and supplements with dosages. Write a brief summary of your goals for DMSO use, being specific about what you hope to achieve.

This preparation serves another crucial function: organizing this information forces you to think clearly about what you're doing and why. If you can't articulate your goals or document your approach in writing, you probably shouldn't be using DMSO yet.

Assembling an Evidence Packet That Builds Credibility

A stack of random internet printouts suggests desperation. A focused evidence packet shows you've engaged with actual research and understand the difference between quality evidence and promotional material.

Start with peer-reviewed studies relevant to your specific condition. If you're using DMSO for knee arthritis, find clinical trials examining topical DMSO for osteoarthritis. PubMed provides free access to abstracts and many full-text articles. Three to five high-quality papers demonstrate you've looked at real research. Print abstracts at minimum, full text if available. Highlight sections describing methods, results, and conclusions. Your doctor can skim these in a minute or two and immediately understands you're referencing legitimate research.

Include a fact sheet summarizing DMSO's legal and regulatory status. Many physicians assume DMSO is illegal or only approved for veterinary use, neither of which is true. A one-page summary stating that DMSO is FDA-approved for interstitial cystitis in humans, widely used off-label for other conditions, and legally available as a pharmaceutical-grade product clears up misconceptions.

Add a safety summary addressing common concerns. Note DMSO's long track record since the 1960s, that serious adverse events are rare when a pharmaceutical-grade product is used appropriately, and the specific safety protocols you're following. Include information about garlic breath so your doctor understands this is a known, harmless phenomenon.

Keep the entire packet under ten pages. Your physician won't read fifty pages, but they will flip through ten well-organized, relevant pages. The evidence packet demonstrates you're approaching DMSO seriously and systematically rather than chasing miracle cures.

Questions That Open Dialogue Rather Than Close It

The questions you ask signal whether you're genuinely seeking input or just looking for permission to do what you've already decided.

"Are there known interactions between DMSO and my current medications?" is specific, shows you understand medication safety importance, and asks about something your physician can answer with confidence. Even if they're not familiar with DMSO specifically, they can identify drug classes that might be concerning with a penetration enhancer.

"Have you had other patients who have tried DMSO for similar conditions?" explores your doctor's experience without putting them on the defensive. If they have encountered DMSO use, you benefit from their observations. If they haven't, the question opens a conversation about whether they'd be willing to supervise your trial.

"What warning signs should I watch for?" positions your provider as the expert on safety monitoring. Physicians think systematically about what could go wrong and what symptoms might indicate problems. It demonstrates you're not blindly committed to DMSO regardless of outcomes.

"Would you be willing to monitor my progress if I proceed with DMSO use?" makes collaboration explicit. Some physicians will decline, preferring not to be involved with therapies outside their comfort zone. Others will agree to monitor even if skeptical, giving you medical oversight.

"What outcomes would convince you this approach is working or not working?" establishes objective criteria for success. By asking what metrics matter to your doctor, you ensure you're tracking data that will be meaningful in future discussions.

Avoid questions that sound accusatory or suggest you've already made up your mind. "Why won't you help me try something natural instead of just prescribing more drugs?" creates conflict. "Don't you think patients should have the right to try alternative approaches?" turns a medical consultation into a political debate.

Setting a Collaborative Tone From the Start

The first words out of your mouth often determine whether the entire conversation will be productive or adversarial.

An effective opening acknowledges your provider's expertise while clearly stating your intention: "I've been researching options for managing my knee pain beyond what we've already tried, and I've come across information about topical DMSO. I know this isn't something you typically recommend, and I wanted to get your input on whether it might be appropriate in my situation and what concerns you might have."

This positions DMSO as one option among many, acknowledges this isn't standard treatment, explicitly seeks your provider's input, and invites them to raise concerns. Be clear about what you're asking for. Are you asking permission? Asking for supervision? Asking for help with monitoring? "What I'm hoping for from this conversation is your assessment of whether DMSO use would interfere with my current medications and whether you'd be willing to monitor my progress if I decide to try it."

The opening tone should be respectful but not apologetic. You don't need to apologize for being interested in DMSO. You're exercising appropriate ownership of your health decisions while seeking expert input.

What to Say When Your Doctor Is Skeptical: Scripts That Work

The theoretical approach to discussing DMSO is one thing. The actual words you use in the moment require more concrete guidance. Having specific language ready prevents you from becoming defensive or inarticulate when the conversation doesn't go smoothly.

Word-for-Word Scripts for Common Scenarios

When your provider has never heard of DMSO, try: "DMSO is dimethyl sulfoxide, a compound that's been used medically since the 1960s. It's FDA-approved for bladder instillation in interstitial cystitis, and it's widely used off-label for pain and inflammation. The research I've found suggests it has anti-inflammatory and analgesic properties when applied topically. I've brought some peer-reviewed studies that show its effects on arthritis pain specifically. Would you be willing to take a look at these and let me know what you think?"

This provides just enough information without overwhelming, establishes legitimacy through FDA approval, acknowledges off-label status, and immediately offers evidence.

When your provider expresses concern about safety, respond with: "I understand your concern about safety. That's actually one of the main reasons I wanted to discuss this with you rather than just trying it on my own. I'm using pharmaceutical-grade DMSO, not industrial grade, and I've researched proper dilution protocols. The main side effect in the literature is skin irritation, which I'm monitoring carefully. What I'd really value from you is guidance on what warning signs would indicate I should stop immediately, and whether you see any specific concerns given my medical history."

This acknowledges their concern as legitimate, demonstrates you've thought about safety seriously, and turns their concern into an opportunity for them to contribute expertise.

If your doctor says they don't feel comfortable recommending DMSO because they're not familiar with it, try: "I completely understand that, and I'm not asking you to recommend something you're not comfortable with. What I'm hoping for is that you'd be willing to monitor me while I try this, even if you're skeptical about whether it will work. I'd like to check in after a month and review how it's going based on objective measures like my pain scores and functional capacity. If you're seeing problems I'm not aware of, or if there's no improvement after a reasonable trial, I'd value your input on whether to continue."

This respects their boundaries while still seeking involvement. It shifts from asking them to endorse DMSO to asking them to observe and assess.

When facing outright dismissal like "That's just snake oil" or "There's no evidence for that," respond with: "I appreciate your skepticism because it keeps me from chasing treatments that don't have support. That's actually why I've brought these peer-reviewed studies from mainstream medical journals. I'm not basing this on testimonials or promotional websites. Would you be willing to look at this research and point out any methodological problems you see? If the studies aren't convincing to you, I'd like to understand why so I can make a better-informed decision."

This validates their skepticism as a professional virtue, reframes the conversation from "you're wrong" to "help me evaluate this evidence," and invites them to use their critical thinking skills.

If your provider suggests prescription alternatives you've already tried, say: "I really appreciate that you're thinking about other options. I've actually tried several of those approaches. The NSAIDs caused stomach problems even with a proton pump inhibitor, and the physical therapy helped initially, but I've plateaued. I'm not looking to replace medical treatment or avoid proven therapies. I'm looking for something additional that might help me reduce my reliance on medications that are causing side effects. Does that make sense given what you know about my treatment history?"

This demonstrates you're not rejecting conventional medicine; you're seeking to augment it based on real limitations you've encountered.

Addressing Different Provider Personalities

The evidence-based physician who values research will respond well to peer-reviewed studies. Focus on the research you've found, acknowledge gaps in evidence, and ask them to evaluate study quality. These providers often respect well-researched approaches and agree to monitor if you present a reasonable protocol.

The clinically conservative physician who prefers proven treatments needs reassurance that you're not abandoning standard care. Emphasize you're looking to add DMSO to your existing treatment plan, not replace evidence-based approaches. Highlight DMSO's long history of use and FDA approval for one indication.

The integrative or holistic physician who's already open to complementary approaches often needs the least convincing. With these providers, you can have more nuanced conversations about the mechanism of action, optimal dosing strategies, and how to integrate DMSO with other treatments.

The time-pressed physician who has seven minutes per patient needs efficiency above all. Have a one-page summary ready covering key points: what DMSO is, why you want to try it, what research supports it, what safety concerns exist, and specifically what you need from them.

Common Objections and How to Address Them

"There isn't enough research to support this" gets addressed with: "You're right that large-scale, recent trials are limited. The research that exists is older and often consists of smaller studies. But what I'm seeing is fairly consistent findings of pain reduction and anti-inflammatory effects with a good safety profile. Given that the alternatives I've tried have had significant side effects or haven't worked well, a therapy with moderate evidence and low risk seems worth trying with proper monitoring. What would you consider adequate evidence to justify a careful trial?"

"I don't know enough about it to advise you" becomes: "I understand that completely, and I'm not expecting you to become a DMSO expert. What would be most helpful is if you could review these few key studies I've brought and let me know if you see red flags I'm missing. And even if you're not advising me to use it, would you be willing to monitor for problems while I try it?"

"This isn't standard of care" gets met with: "You're absolutely right that it's not standard treatment. I've tried the standard approaches, including NSAIDs and physical therapy. I'm looking at DMSO as an additional option for managing symptoms that haven't fully responded to standard care. Does it make sense to try this as an adjunct rather than a replacement?"

Closing with an Invitation for Ongoing Collaboration

How you end the conversation matters as much as how you begin it. Try this closing: "I really appreciate you taking the time to discuss this with me. Based on our conversation, here's what I'm proposing: I'll start with a very conservative protocol using low-concentration DMSO, tracking my symptoms daily, and monitoring for any side effects. I'd like to check back with you in four weeks to review how it's going. Would you be open to helping me track my results and adjust the protocol as needed?"

Another effective closing: "What warning signs should I specifically watch for and report to you? I want to make sure I'm monitoring the right things and that I contact you immediately if concerning symptoms develop. Should I keep a log of pain levels and any side effects to bring to my next appointment?"

If they remain skeptical but agree to monitor: "I hear that you're not convinced this will work, and you may be right. What I appreciate is your willingness to supervise this trial and help me evaluate objectively whether it's beneficial. Let's agree on specific outcomes that would indicate success or failure. What metrics would you want to see improve for this to be worthwhile?"

After the Appointment: Creating Your DMSO Care Plan and Tracking System

You've prepared your evidence, practiced your scripts, and successfully navigated the conversation. Now comes transforming that initial dialogue into an ongoing collaborative relationship built on systematic documentation and clear communication.

You're the Hub: Becoming Your Own Care Coordinator

DMSO doesn't exist in isolation from the rest of your healthcare. You likely have multiple providers managing different aspects of your health. Adding DMSO without coordination creates gaps where important interactions or contraindications slip through unnoticed.

Integrated care means everyone involved in your health knows what everyone else is doing. Your rheumatologist understands you're using topical DMSO and can factor that into their assessment. Your physical therapist knows you apply DMSO before sessions and can time their manual therapy accordingly. Your pharmacist has a complete picture of everything you're taking and can flag potential interactions. You become the central coordinator, ensuring information flows between these separate spheres of care.

Documenting Your Approach: What Every Provider Needs to See

Verbal communication about DMSO use fails too often. You mention you're using DMSO, your doctor makes a note about "some topical treatment," and six months later, they have no idea what you're actually doing. Written documentation solves this.

Create a DMSO protocol document specifying exactly what you're doing. Include the concentration (stated as a percentage and what you dilute with, for example, "60% DMSO in aloe vera gel"), frequency of application (how many times daily and which days per week), body locations where you apply DMSO, the amount you use per application, and your monitoring steps.

Add a brief statement of your goals. "Reduce knee pain by 50% to allow increased walking and stair climbing without assistance" is specific and measurable. Update this document whenever you change your protocol and redistribute it to your care team so everyone has current information.

Share this document with every provider involved in your care: your primary care doctor, any specialists, your pharmacist, and any complementary practitioners. Don't assume they'll communicate with each other.

Turning Daily Logs into Doctor-Friendly Summaries

Basic tracking creates the foundation. Now transform that raw daily data into professional presentations that give providers actionable information.

Raw data dumps overwhelm busy healthcare providers. Organized summaries highlighting key trends generate useful feedback. Before appointments, create a progress summary covering the reporting period since your last visit. Include your average pain levels for the period, the number of DMSO applications you completed versus what you planned (showing compliance rate), any protocol changes you made and when, and notable improvements or setbacks.

A one-page summary covering four weeks of daily tracking gives your provider digestible information rather than 28 pages of raw logs. Simple visualizations communicate trends faster than columns of numbers. A hand-drawn graph showing pain levels over time, with notation of when you started DMSO or increased concentration, tells the story at a glance.

Highlight positive trends explicitly: "My average pain decreased from 7.5 out of 10 to 4.5 over this four-week period," or "I increased my walking distance from one block to four blocks." Equally important, identify plateaus and setbacks clearly: "Pain improvement plateaued at 5 out of 10 after the second week," or "I had a flare-up in week three that increased pain back to 7."

Connect outcomes to specific protocol elements when your data reveals these relationships: "Pain reduction was most significant during the two weeks when I used 70% concentration twice daily," or "I experienced increased skin irritation when I switched from aloe to water as a carrier, which resolved when I switched back."

Providers need to see certain key metrics: average pain levels over time showing whether you're improving, stable, or worsening; compliance rates showing applications completed versus planned; functional improvements like walking distance or range of motion; and side effects and how you managed them.

Ask for specific feedback based on your data: "Based on these results, do you think I should continue at this concentration or adjust?" or "The plateau I hit at week three concerns me. Does this suggest I've reached maximum benefit from DMSO, or might a different protocol help?"

Your Pharmacist Is an Expert Too: Getting Interaction Advice

Pharmacists are underutilized resources. They have extensive training in drug interactions and typically have more time to discuss medications than physicians during brief appointments.

Schedule a consultation with your pharmacist specifically to discuss DMSO interactions with your current medications and supplements. Bring a complete list of everything you take, including prescription medications with dosages, over-the-counter medications, and all supplements. Include your DMSO protocol document.

Ask specific questions: "Are any of my medications likely to have altered absorption if I'm using DMSO topically?" and "How long should I wait before applying prescription creams to other body areas after using DMSO?" Ask your pharmacist to flag medications in your profile that would require stopping DMSO if prescribed in the future.

Who's Watching What: Defining Oversight Responsibilities

When multiple providers are involved, confusion about who's overseeing what creates dangerous gaps. Explicitly clarify roles.

Identify a point person for DMSO oversight, typically your primary care physician, since they co-ordinate your overall care. Make this explicit by asking directly whether they're comfortable serving this role. Schedule regular check-ins for protocol review built into existing visits rather than requiring separate appointments. Establish a clear process for updating all providers when you change your protocol. Document who monitors which aspects of your health in relation to DMSO use.

Beyond Doctor Visits: Using Data to Optimize Your Own Protocol

Provider communication represents one valuable use of tracking data, but personal insight and autonomous optimization may be equally important.

Review your logs weekly, looking for patterns. Do certain activities predictably increase your pain regardless of DMSO use, suggesting you need activity modification? Does your pain vary with weather, stress levels, or sleep quality in ways DMSO can't overcome? Do you see correlations between DMSO application timing and pain relief duration? These patterns emerge only through systematic review.

Look for triggers that undermine DMSO's effectiveness. If your logs show pain spikes on days when you eat certain foods, sleep poorly, or experience high stress, DMSO alone won't solve your problem.

Use your data to conduct personal experiments. Try morning versus evening applications for two weeks each while tracking results systematically. Compare the daily application to every other day to find your minimum effective frequency. Test different concentrations methodically, changing only one variable at a time. Experiment with different carriers to discover which produces the best results with the least irritation.

Set a calendar reminder for the first Sunday of each month to conduct a formal monthly review. Spend 15 to 20 minutes summarizing the past four weeks of data. Calculate your average pain level for the month and compare it to previous months. Identify whether you're improving, plateauing, or worsening. Look for protocol changes that correlate with shifts in outcomes. Plan your protocol adjustments for the coming month based on what you're learning.

Tracking also reveals when DMSO has reached its limits. If improvement plateaus for two or more months despite systematic protocol adjustments, you've likely extracted the maximum benefit DMSO can provide. This isn't failure; it's valuable information. Some people achieve 30% improvement with DMSO, others 70%, and tracking shows which category you fall into.

Your tracking data might also reveal that factors beyond DMSO control significantly impact your symptoms. If stress, sleep quality, or physical activity patterns show stronger correlations with your pain than DMSO concentration or frequency, that information guides you toward interventions addressing those factors.

Finally, use tracking as a self-advocacy tool to build evidence for additional interventions you might need. If your data clearly shows DMSO reduces your pain from 7 to 4, but you need to reach 2 for adequate function, this documented partial response supports requesting physical therapy, medication adjustment, or specialist referral. Providers respond far more favorably to data-driven requests than to subjective complaints unsupported by objective evidence.

Keeping the Healing Going

Now that you have what you need to use DMSO safely and confidently for pain relief, joint support, muscle recovery, and inflammation, it's time to pass this knowledge forward.

By leaving your honest review on Amazon, you help other readers who are searching for natural ways to feel better find this book and get the guidance they need.

Your words may be the reason someone finally finds relief, hope, and a simple path forward.

Simply scan the QR code or click the link below to leave your review:

https://www.amazon.com/review/review-your-purchases/?asin=B0GWWLW4JM

Thank you for your support. The power of DMSO continues to grow when we share what we learn, and you are helping make that possible.

Printable Bonuses

Quick Reference Guides

Bonus #1: DMSO Concentration Quick Reference Chart

Bonus #2: Carrier Comparison Chart

Bonus #3: Safety Rules One-Pager

Bonus #4: Emergency Response Card

Printable Templates and Worksheets

Bonus #5: Daily DMSO Application Log

Bonus #6: Symptom Tracking Worksheet

Bonus #7: Monthly Review Worksheet

Bonus #8: Progress Summary Template (for Doctor Visits)

Decision Support Tools

Bonus #9: "Should I Use DMSO?" Decision Tree

Bonus #10: Concentration Selection Flowchart

Bonus #11: Troubleshooting Decision Tree

Safety Checklists

Bonus #12: Pre-Application Safety Checklist

Bonus #13: Product Quality Verification Checklist

Bonus #14: Skin Preparation Checklist

Communiction Tools

Bonus #15: DMSO Protocol Document Template (for Providers)

Bonus #16: Doctor Conversation Script

Bonus #17: Pharmacist Consultation Script

Bonus #18: Evidence Packet Template

Recipes and Formulas

Bonus #19: Recipe Cards for Common Blends

Action Guides

Bonus #20: Quick Start Guide (First 5 Steps with DMSO)

Bonus #21: Product Sourcing Guide (Where to Buy Safely)

To Download the Bonuses, please scan the QR code or click on the link below:

https://tinyurl.com/2u3yn5vk

Conclusion

Your DMSO Journey Starts Here

You made it. You've read through the science, the safety protocols, the practical applications, and the advanced strategies. You understand what DMSO is, how it works, and what it can and cannot do. You know how to choose quality products, dilute them safely, and apply them correctly. You have checklists, decision trees, tracking logs, and conversation scripts. You're equipped.

But here's what I want you to remember most: this book is a starting point, not a finish line.

DMSO is not going to work the same way for you as it does for your neighbor, your friend, or the person who recommended it to you. Your body is different. Your condition is different. Your tolerance, your skin sensitivity, your response to treatment, all of it is uniquely yours. And that means your DMSO protocol needs to be uniquely yours too.

The most important skill you've gained from this book is not memorizing concentration percentages or knowing which carrier works best for knee pain. It is knowing how to experiment responsibly. How to start small, track systematically, adjust methodically, and recognize when something is working or when it is time to try something different.

What Success Really Looks Like

If you are like most people starting with DMSO, you are hoping for one thing: relief. You want less pain, better mobility, and fewer limitations. And DMSO might give you that. For some people, the results are dramatic. They go from a pain level of 8 to a 3 within weeks. They are back to activities they had given up on. They feel like they got their life back.

For others, the improvement is more modest. A reduction from 7 to 5. Enough to sleep better at night, but not enough to eliminate the problem. And for a smaller group, DMSO does not move the needle much at all.

All three of those outcomes are valid data. They all tell you something important about your body and your condition. Even if DMSO only gets you partway there, that partial response might be exactly what you need to layer in other interventions such as physical therapy, medication adjustments, and lifestyle changes, and finally achieve the relief you are looking for.

Success with DMSO is not measured by how many symptoms disappear. It is measured by how much clearer you are about what your body needs.

The Most Common Mistakes (and How to Avoid Them)

As you start your DMSO journey, watch out for these traps:

Mistake #1: **Starting too strong**. You are in pain. You want relief now. So you jump straight to 80% concentration twice a day because you assume more must be better. Then your skin reacts, you get discouraged, and you quit before giving DMSO a real chance. Start low. Build slowly. Give your skin and your body time to adapt.

Mistake #2: **Inconsistency**. You use DMSO for three days, feel a little better, and stop. Then your pain comes back, so you restart. Then you get busy and forget for a week. DMSO works best with consistent use. If you are going to try it, commit to at least 2 to 4 weeks of daily application before you decide whether it is helping.

Mistake #3: **Ignoring your data**. You are tracking pain levels, applications, and side effects in your log, but you never actually look at the patterns. The whole point of tracking is to learn. Set aside 15 minutes at the end of each week to review what is working and what is not. Adjust based on evidence, not guesswork.

Mistake #4: **Going it alone**. You do not tell your doctor. You do not ask your pharmacist about interactions. You assume you can figure it all out by yourself. DMSO is generally safe, but it is not risk free. Bring your healthcare team into the conversation. They can help you spot problems early and integrate DMSO into your overall care plan.

What to Do When DMSO Is Not Enough

Let's say you have done everything right. You have used DMSO consistently for two months. You have tracked your results carefully. You have adjusted your concentration, tried different carriers, and experimented with timing. And you have plateaued at a 30% improvement. You are better than you were, but you are still not where you need to be.

This is not failure. This is information.

DMSO has shown you it can help, just not all the way. Now you know you are a partial responder. That tells your doctor something valuable. It tells them your condition is responsive to anti inflammatory treatment, which means other anti inflammatory interventions might also help. It tells them your pain is not purely structural or nerve related. It gives them a starting point for figuring out what else to try.

Use your DMSO data as a foundation for building a more comprehensive treatment plan. If DMSO got you from 7 to 5, what else can bridge that gap from 5 to 2? Physical therapy? Dietary changes? A different medication? A combination approach?

DMSO does not have to be your only tool. It just has to be a useful one.

The Power of Taking Back Control

Here is what I hope you take away from this book more than anything else: you are not powerless.

For too long, you have probably felt like pain is something that happens to you. Something you endure. Something you manage with whatever tools your doctor gives you, hoping they will work.

But DMSO puts you back in the driver's seat. You get to decide when to apply it, where to apply it, and how much to use. You get to track the results. You get to adjust the protocol. You get to experiment, learn, and refine.

This is active participation in your own health. Not passive acceptance. Not blind hope. Not resignation.

And even if DMSO ends up being just one piece of your pain management puzzle, the skills you have learned here, how to track symptoms, how to experiment systematically, how to communicate with providers, and how to interpret your own data, those skills transfer to everything else you try.

You are not just learning about DMSO. You are learning how to take ownership of your healing.

Moving Forward: Your First 30 Days

If you are ready to start, here is what I recommend for your first month:

Week 1: Complete the "Should I Use DMSO?" decision tree (Bonus #9). If you pass all the safety screens, order pharmaceutical grade DMSO and perform your 24 hour patch test. Read through the Pre Application Safety Checklist (Bonus #12) and the Skin Preparation Checklist (Bonus #14) until you can do them from memory.

Week 2: Start with the lowest recommended concentration for your application area (see Bonus #1). Apply once daily. Track every single application in your Daily DMSO Application Log (Bonus #5). Do not change anything yet, just collect data.

Week 3: Review your first week of data using the Weekly Summary Worksheet (Bonus #6). Are you seeing any improvement? Any side effects? Based on what you are learning, make one small adjustment if needed, either increase concentration by 10% or add a second daily application. Continue tracking.

Week 4: Complete your Monthly Review Worksheet (Bonus #7). Calculate your average pain reduction. Assess whether your current protocol is working or whether you need to make further adjustments. Decide whether to continue, modify, or stop.

After 30 days, you will have real data. Not hunches. Not guesses. Evidence. And evidence is what gives you the power to make truly informed decisions about what comes next.

A Final Word

I wrote this book because I believe you deserve better than vague advice, scare tactics, and false promises. You deserve clear information, practical tools, and the respect to make your own choices.

DMSO is not magic. It will not cure everything. It will not work perfectly for everyone.

But for many people, it offers something incredibly valuable: meaningful relief without the side effects, costs, or risks of pharmaceutical alternatives. A chance to move more freely, sleep more soundly, and reclaim activities that pain had taken away.

Whether DMSO becomes a cornerstone of your pain management or just a helpful tool you use occasionally, you now have the knowledge to use it safely, effectively, and intelligently.

The power is in your hands, literally.

Track your results. Listen to your body. Adjust as needed. And do not be afraid to experiment within the boundaries of safety.

Your relief is out there. Sometimes it takes a little trial and error to find it. But you are equipped now. You know what to do.

Welcome to the beginning of your DMSO journey. I am honored to have been part of it.

Here is to less pain, more freedom, and taking back control.

You have got this.

Resources

Agarwal, R., Iezhitsa, I., Agarwal, P., Abdul Nasir, N. A., Razali, N., Alyautdin, R., & Ismail, N. M. (2016). Liposomes in topical ophthalmic drug delivery: An update. Drug Delivery, 23(4), 1075–1091. https://doi.org/10.3109/10717544.2014.943336

Bastos, C. R., & Pereira, M. L. (2017). Dimethyl sulfoxide (DMSO) in acute ischemic stroke. Cochrane Database of Systematic Reviews, 2017(9), Article CD009585. https://doi.org/10.1002/14651858.CD009585.pub2

Blythe, L. L., Gilete, N. A., Jacobson, J. K., & Craig, A. M. (1986). Effect of transportation, handling, and dimethylsulfoxide on plasma alpha-tocopherol in horses. American Journal of Veterinary Research, 47(11), 2187–2189.

Brayton, C. F. (1986). Dimethyl sulfoxide (DMSO): A review. Cornell Veterinarian, 76(1), 61–90.

Burgess, D. J., Kwok, K. K., & Megremis, P. T. (1991). Characterization of albumin microspheres by light scattering. Pharmaceutical Research, 8(12), 1548–1553. https://doi.org/10.1023/A:1015805812261

Capriotti, K., & Capriotti, J. A. (2012). Dimethyl sulfoxide: History, chemistry, and clinical utility in dermatology. The Journal of Clinical and Aesthetic Dermatology, 5(9), 24–26.

David, N. A. (1972). The pharmacology of dimethyl sulfoxide. Annual Review of Pharmacology, 12, 353–374. https://doi.org/10.1146/annurev.pa.12.040172.002033

Eberhardt, R., Zwingers, T., & Hofmann, R. (1990). DMSO in patients with active gonarthrosis: A double-blind placebo controlled phase III study. Fortschritte der Medizin, 108(27), 534–538.

Elisia, I., Nakamura, H., Lam, V., Hofs, E., Cederberg, R., Cait, J., Hughes, M. R., Lee, L., Jia, W., Adomat, H. H., Guns, E. S. T., McNagny, K. M., & Krystal, G. (2016). DMSO represses inflammatory cytokine production from human blood cells and reduces autoimmune arthritis. PLOS ONE, 11(3), Article e0152538. https://doi.org/10.1371/journal.pone.0152538

Engelhardt, J. A. (1998). Comparative renal toxicopathology of anticancer agents. Toxicologic Pathology, 26(1), 18–30. https://doi.org/10.1177/019262339802600103

Evans, M. S., Reid, K. H., & Sharp, J. B., Jr. (1993). Dimethylsulfoxide (DMSO) blocks conduction in peripheral nerve C fibers: A possible mechanism of analgesia. Neuroscience Letters, 150(2), 145–148. https://doi.org/10.1016/0304-3940(93)90523-t

Gordon, D. M. (1967). Dimethyl sulfoxide in ophthalmology, with special reference to possible toxic effects. Archives of Ophthalmology, 78(4), 447–449. https://doi.org/10.1001/archopht.1967.00980030449006

Gurtner, G. C., & Wong, V. W. (2013). Dimethyl sulfoxide. In Wound healing: A paradigm for regeneration (pp. 367–378). Elsevier.

Jacob, S. W., & Herschler, R. (1986). Pharmacology of DMSO. Cryobiology, 23(1), 14–27. https://doi.org/10.1016/0011-2240(86)90014-3

Jacob, S. W., & Rosenbaum, E. E. (1971). The biological actions and medical applications of dimethyl sulfoxide. Annals of the New York Academy of Sciences, Vol. 141, Article 1.

Jacob, S. W., & Wood, D. C. (1967). Dimethyl sulfoxide (DMSO): Toxicology, pharmacology, and clinical experience. American Journal of Surgery, 114(3), 414–426. https://doi.org/10.1016/0002-9610(67)90017-2

Jacob, S. W., Lawrence, R. M., & Zucker, M. (2009). The miracle of MSM: The natural solution for pain. Berkley Books.

Jimenez, R. A., & Willkens, R. F. (1967). Dimethyl sulfoxide: A perspective of its use in rheumatic diseases. Journal of Laboratory and Clinical Medicine, 70(4), 659–672.

Kollerup Madsen, B., Hilscher, M., Zetner, D., & Rosenberg, J. (2018). Adverse reactions of dimethyl sulfoxide in humans: A systematic review. F1000Research, 7, Article 1746. https://doi.org/10.12688/f1000research.16642.2

Marren, K. (2011). Dimethyl sulfoxide: An effective penetration enhancer for topical administration of NSAIDs. The Physician and Sportsmedicine, 39(3), 75–82. https://doi.org/10.3810/psm.2011.09.1923

Morton, J. I., & Siegel, B. V. (1986). Effects of oral dimethyl sulfoxide and dimethyl sulfone on murine autoimmune lymphoproliferative disease. Proceedings of the Society for Experimental Biology and Medicine, 183(2), 227–230. https://doi.org/10.3181/00379727-183-42409

Murav'ev, I. V., Venikova, M. S., Pleskovskaia, G. N., Riazantseva, T. A., & Sigidin, I. A. (1991). Effect of dimethyl sulfoxide and dimethyl sulfone on a destructive process in the joints of mice with spontaneous arthritis. Patologicheskaia Fiziologiia i Eksperimental'naia Terapiia, (2), 37–39.

National Center for Biotechnology Information. (2024). PubChem compound summary for CID 679, Dimethyl sulfoxide. https://pubchem.ncbi.nlm.nih.gov/compound/Dimethyl-sulfoxide

National Institutes of Health, National Library of Medicine. (n.d.). DailyMed: RIMSO-50 (dimethyl sulfoxide) solution. https://dailymed.nlm.nih.gov/

Penrod, L. E., & Newman, H. C. (1966). Dimethyl sulfoxide in musculoskeletal disorders. Canadian Medical Association Journal, 94(22), 1179–1181.

Perkins, N. R., & Threlfall, W. R. (2013). Dimethylsulfoxide: Its use in large animal practice. Veterinary Clinics of North America: Equine Practice, 29(3), 663–676.

Ramadan, M. A., Shawkey, A. E., Rabeh, M. A., & Abdellatif, A. O. (2019). Expression of P-glycoprotein in retinal tissues of streptozotocin-induced diabetic rats and its modulation by fenofibrate and crocin. Biomedicine & Pharmacotherapy, 110, 652–659. https://doi.org/10.1016/j.biopha.2018.12.012

Salim, S. (2017). Oxidative stress and the central nervous system. Journal of Pharmacology and Experimental Therapeutics, 360(1), 201–205. https://doi.org/10.1124/jpet.116.237503

Santos, N. C., Figueira-Coelho, J., Martins-Silva, J., & Saldanha, C. (2003). Multidisciplinary utilization of dimethyl sulfoxide: Pharmacological, cellular, and molecular aspects. Biochemical Pharmacology, 65(7), 1035–1041. https://doi.org/10.1016/s0006-2952(03)00002-9

Shirley, S. W., Stewart, B. H., & Mirelman, S. (1978). Dimethyl sulfoxide in treatment of inflammatory genitourinary disorders. Urology, 11(3), 215–220. https://doi.org/10.1016/0090-4295(78)90057-7

Swanson, B. N. (1985). Medical use of dimethyl sulfoxide (DMSO). Reviews of Clinical & Basic Pharmacology, 5(1–2), 1–33.

Toxic Substances Control Act (TSCA) Chemical Substance Inventory. U.S. Environmental Protection Agency. (2024). Dimethyl sulfoxide (CAS 67-68-5). https://www.epa.gov/tsca-inventory

U.S. Food and Drug Administration. (1978). Dimethyl sulfoxide (DMSO) approval for interstitial cystitis [Drug approval package]. U.S. Department of Health and Human Services.

U.S. Food and Drug Administration. (2024). Drugs@FDA: FDA-approved drugs. https://www.accessdata.fda.gov/scripts/cder/daf/

U.S. Food and Drug Administration, Center for Veterinary Medicine. (n.d.). Approved animal drug products (Green Book). https://www.fda.gov/animal-veterinary/approved-animal-drug-products-green-book

Williams, H. J., Furst, D. E., Dahl, S. L., Steen, V. D., Marks, C., Alpert, E. J., Furst, B., Majerus, T., Beatty, J. G., & Green, F. A. (1985). Double-blind, multicenter controlled trial comparing topical dimethyl sulfoxide and normal saline for treatment of hand ulcers in patients with systemic sclerosis. Arthritis & Rheumatism, 28(3), 308–314. https://doi.org/10.1002/art.1780280311

Yu, Z. W., & Quinn, P. J. (1994). Dimethyl sulphoxide: A review of its applications in cell biology. Bioscience Reports, 14(6), 259–281. https://doi.org/10.1007/BF01199051

Made in the USA
Monee, IL
16 September 2026

62980087R00070